BETWEEN

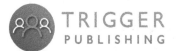

TRIGGER
PUBLISHING

ABOUT THE AUTHORS

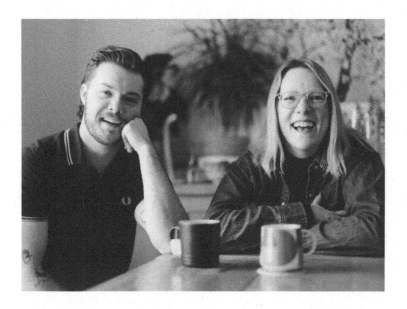

Leo Telford is a 21-year-old trans man and student at the University of East Anglia, studying sociology, with a view to going into teaching. Leo has A-levels in sociology, politics and business.

Gemma Telford is a 52-year-old parent of a trans son and self-employed marketing consultant who has worked for more than 20 years in the technology industry, helping technology businesses go to market in the UK, Europe and globally.

Visit Leo and Gemma's website: www.betweenbook.co.uk

BETWEEN

A memoir on gender transition by a
mother and her trans son

BY GEMMA AND LEO TELFORD

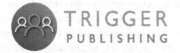

Published in 2025 by Trigger Publishing
An imprint of Shaw Callaghan Ltd

UK Office
The Stanley Building
7 Pancras Square
Kings Cross
London N1C 4AG

US Office
On Point Executive Center, Inc
3030 N Rocky Point Drive W
Suite 150
Tampa, FL 33607
www.triggerpublishing.com

A CIP catalogue record for this book is available upon
request from the British Library
ISBN: 978-1-83796-084-2
eBook ISBN: 978-1-83796-085-9

Cover design by Francesca Corsini
Typeset by Lapiz Digital Services

CONTENTS

A NOTE FROM LEO AND GEMMA

For the purposes of this book and to help it make sense, we've decided that we're going to refer to Leo as E, the initial of his birth name, during the period that he was this person to our family. We understand that many transgender people never want to use/be associated with their birth name (or "deadname", as it's often called). We totally respect that, but Leo is okay with us using his initial instead of his name in this book to help to make sense of the story.

We also wanted to explain why Leo's dad and brothers don't feature more in the book. That's because it's our story – we chose to write it and we chose what to share about our experiences. Leo's dad, and his younger brother especially, are mentioned in the book in some sections, but don't want to be a big feature and have asked not to be a part of it in the same way. Not because they don't absolutely love and support Leo's transition – we all want to be clear that they really do – but because their feelings are their feelings, and we can only write the book about our own experiences. Luca, Leo's younger brother, was very young when Leo first came out, and so a lot of the difficult period we went through didn't affect him in quite the same way. Likewise, Bill, Leo's dad, has never been a great talker and found much of the process we went through very difficult. He was happy for the book to be from just our point of view, and so it is.

We know, sadly from experience, that some people may "blame" some of what we have gone through on a perceived lack of a father figure in his life. That is not and has never been the case. Leo's dad has always been a huge influence and support to Leo, and he continues to be. Leo has parents who are happily married and have been for over 20 years. Leo comes from a secure and loving family. So there, haters.

INTRODUCTION

Gemma

E was never a very girly girl, but it didn't seem to matter too much. After all, I'd been a tomboy too – often mistaken for a boy, especially in my pre-teen years. So what if people thought E was a boy? As a feminist, I tried not to impose gender stereotypes on either of my kids and wanted them both to believe they could achieve anything they set their minds to. Gender didn't have to get in the way.

Sometimes I noticed a gender bias in myself I hadn't been aware of though. E wanted a football shirt, and I didn't want her to wear one ... although I was okay with my son, Luca, doing so. She wanted to wear boys' clothes and pretty much refused to wear girls' clothes. That was okay, but it was frustrating that she wouldn't even wear plain T-shirts in blue or red, just because they were from the girls' range.

Looking back now, of course, the signs were there. My child was transgender. When she was three or four, she was insistent that she was a boy – and wanted us to call her "John Lewis" (like the shop!). It was a family joke for years. But what I didn't realize until almost a decade later was that, in fact, that was her earliest expression of who she was. E really did see herself as a boy, and as soon as she was able to tell the difference, she did.

This is a story of journeys, personal growth, relationships, coming to terms with loss, challenges and heartbreak, but also of reflection, love and family. It's a story about how our daughter became our son.

For me, becoming a parent came with the utter shock of love in the early days, mixed in with fear, anxiety and a constant worry about doing the right thing. Any parent knows the feeling of watching your kids grow up and change and wondering, *Are you doing the best for them, for yourself? What even is your best?* Some days it's as much as you can do just to get through the day and make it to bedtime – theirs and yours! And every parent has had to face things their child has done that they haven't liked, or what that's meant they've done because of, or in response to that action. We're all fallible. We are all learning all the time. And sometimes we really fuck things up.

This book is not supposed to be some kind of heart-warming tale about how love overcomes any challenge you can face – although I guess it does in the end (spoiler alert). It's not trying to tell anyone the "right" way to deal with a transgender child because we certainly didn't get it right. It's just my experience of having one. And Leo's experience of being one. Sometimes it went amazingly, heart-burstingly right. And many times, it was just bloody awful and heartbreakingly wrong. It's part therapy and part just sharing a story of being a parent that I hope will have parallels with many other parents, whatever their own kids have gone/are going/will go through.

In this book we've both tried to fairly portray our experiences of organizations and services we've come across and with which we've had dealings. It's not intended to pass judgement or criticize. I recognize that everyone has different experiences, and everyone's experience is unique. All I can do is share my own experience. All Leo can do is share his.

It's also important to stress that just because my child is transgender, I most certainly am not an expert in transgender issues in any way. I know something about it obviously and have read more, tried to educate myself and behave in a way that respects the lived experience of others, including my son. But I won't always have got everything right. So, apologies in advance to anyone for any inaccuracies. Please don't take my words as fact – please do your own research. Speak and listen to transgender people and try to understand what it's really like for them. Be open-minded and open-hearted. Be compassionate.

* * *

Leo

We live in a time in which everyone has heard something about transgender people, whether it's a celebrity coming out, controversy over where we go to the toilet, or discussion about whether trans people should be allowed to compete in sports as the gender they are. Because of all these opinions and the overload of information, the lives of transgender people have been reduced to a talking point, which has, in turn, given the community something of an otherworldly quality for many. What contributes even more to this is the fact that, speaking in terms of probability, most people don't know a trans person first-hand.

For the past few years, there has been an incessant focus on trans people in the media, with newspapers and online media outlets publishing multiple stories each day. But amongst all the debates and opinion-driven reporting, trans people are nowhere to be seen in the conversation. As trans author Shon Faye writes, whilst the visibility of trans people is increasing and greater than ever, it can act as a double-edged sword.[1] On the rare occasion there is a trans person present in a media context, they're often on daytime TV, pitted against a personality such as Piers Morgan, whose desire isn't to inform and educate the public of the hardships and realities of the minority, but to ridicule, reproach and isolate for the purposes of entertainment and divisiveness. Still, as I said before, we struggle when trans people aren't in the picture, too. When that happens, we are reduced to an idea, one that is formulated from misinformation and the product of a moral panic.

Many people are unaware that the transgender community in the UK makes up less than one per cent of the population. (In fact, of the people answering the question on gender identity in the 2021 UK census, just 0.5 per cent said their gender identity and sex registered at birth were different).[2] The reason this isn't a well-known fact is because the way and frequency with which trans people appear in the media magnifies the size of the community and exaggerates our presence in society. Often, innocent ignorance of trans issues means people form their opinions and ideas of what a trans person is based on the media they consume, rather than seeking information from informed sources, or from trans people in real life. This doesn't mean any trans person you might know of or come across is the most suitable person to direct your burning questions to, but the world is home to thousands of trans content creators, authors and online personalities that discuss such things and can share varied and genuine experiences from the community and themselves.

A key misconception I've come across that is the result of reporting on trans children and their social and physical transitions is how unrealistic and over-simplified such processes have been made to appear. It is assumed that it is possible for a child to wake up one day, come out as trans, hop straight onto hormones or puberty blockers with no resistance from NHS agencies, their carers or the law, and it's as easy as that. This couldn't be further from the experience I had, nor from the reality I know my friends and so many young trans people face.

These examples contribute to the reason my mum and I have wanted to share our story. Though the idea first cropped up around seven or eight years ago, watching the discourse and conversation around trans people increasingly become poisoned with misinformation, bias and ignorance led us to decide that now is the right time for a story like ours to be out there. And after the idea had lingered in our heads for years, we feel we are now in the best place we could be in to write this book. With this in mind, we want *Between* to be an open and raw account of the experience a family goes through after a child comes out as transgender. It's a story for someone who is going through the same thing and wants something to relate to, to know they're not alone in the discomfort, anguish and confusing moments. It's also something that people can hopefully learn from. For myself, I want the publication of my experiences to combat the media-manufactured moral panic about trans people and put reality back into the conversation. But above all, *Between* is for anyone who's curious about our situation or of trans people generally and wants something to help them feel informed, or even just for those who were intrigued by the cover. No matter why you've picked up this book, we're glad you're here.

Chapter 1

COMING OUT

Gemma

Is it just me that always had problems putting their kids to bed? When I had E, I was a bit older for a first-time mum at 32. I'd got a good job and thought that because I'd done lots of reading and research, gone to my antenatal classes and made plans, everything would be okay. Spoiler alert – it wasn't!

When I got home from hospital with E, I wondered why no one had really told me about the sleep. Oh God, the sleep ... or lack of it! Probably through my own stress, E never went to sleep easily or stayed asleep. I'm sure it was me transmitting my own tension to her that made it hard for her to relax, but after feeding, rocking and singing, when her eyes eventually closed and I put her down in her cot as gently as physically possible, she would instantly spring awake, crying. I absolutely hated the sound of her crying, and so "letting her cry it out" was never an option for me. I would pick her up and start the process all over again. She would wake up typically three or four times a night, every night. And it didn't get better at three months. Or at six months. In fact, four years later, when we had her baby brother, it *still* wasn't better. At that point, through sheer exhaustion, I asked for help from a health visitor, a community nurse trained specifically to improve the health and wellbeing of families with young children. By this time, E understood the concept of going to bed, and had been out of a cot and in her little bed for two years. But going to sleep and staying asleep was still a problem. And of course, by then I had another newborn who was also waking up! Thankfully, he was easier to get to sleep (although another three months of pain and shame and still not being able to breastfeed saw me dusting off the breast pump again). The health visitor showed me how I could sit next to E while she went to sleep, then sit on the floor, then by the door. Eventually I was sitting outside her door, then on the stairs, and then she could self-settle. So, I only had sleepless nights for the first five years! I know people smile knowingly at new parents and chuckle about sleepless nights, but it really is no joke. I wasn't a stay-at-home mum either – I worked while I had both children. I was lucky that my husband spent the first year of E's life mainly at home to be with her while I worked, and he's always done the school runs. But I always did the nights, as I just couldn't sleep when one of them was crying.

It's safe to say, then, that bedtimes had always been somewhat stressful for E and me. I always wanted to be the one that put my children in bed though, the one who read the story, sang the songs and stroked their hair as they fell asleep. But some nights, bedtime would just get dragged out and out with "one more thing" they "just had to do ...". I'm sure if you're a parent, you'll be familiar with bedtime-delaying tactics. The absolute worst thing at bedtime is when one of your kids gets upset. Sometimes they were upset because I had got snappy because I wanted bedtime to be done. Sometimes it's only in the last minutes of the day that they decide to tell you something important, or something they're worried about. I didn't always handle it well. I was often frazzled, exhausted and desperate to get to bed myself! So, on the night E dropped the bombshell, it was just another frustrating bedtime for me. How I handled (or rather, didn't handle) our conversation that first night is still a deep source of pain and regret for me. And even though Leo has forgiven me for it, I'm not sure I'll ever be able to get over it myself.

On the night in question, E was 11. Bedtimes were usually easier by now, although they were sometimes still dragged out. And because they happened later in the evening than they did when E was little, they cut more into my own downtime when they did get stretched. It was about 9pm one night and we were going through a "normal" night-time routine – brushing teeth (*Come on!*), putting pyjamas on (*It's past your bedtime!*), getting into bed. E started to cry. Just quietly at first, and then more seriously. My first reaction was frustration (*Now you decide to start crying?! Really? There is a glass of wine waiting for me downstairs!*). I passed her a tissue and asked in a clipped, frustrated voice, "What's wrong?" (which probably sounded more like, 'And what's wrong *now*?!'). No answer, so with a big sigh, I sat back down on E's bed and passed some more tissues. Bedtime tears were not normally like this, so although I was still frustrated, I was also now starting to worry. (And when I worry, I also get short and snappy. It's not my best feature and one I can't seem to shift, even now. Worry for me quickly turns into anger and frustration because I feel out of control and unable to help. Even knowing that, it still happens.)

Eventually I realized that snapping was not going to help. I hated seeing E upset and so I asked what was wrong. I stroked the hair away from her red face. I needed to be able to solve whatever the problem was and I was already thinking about it. I told her, "Nothing can be that bad. If you don't tell me what's wrong, how can I help?" What I really meant was, "How can I fix it?" I wasn't taking the time to listen or leaving the space for E to talk. I was just trying to fix a problem by essentially bullying it out of her, so I could provide a simple solution, dry her tears and get downstairs to my wine. The answer I eventually got was not one I expected to hear in a million years.

"Mum, I think I'm a boy."

Stunned silence.

"Oh E, don't be silly. You're not a boy."

Years afterwards, we talked about this moment. How, with one simple sentence, I swept aside all the worry, hurt and anxiety E had gone through up to that point. How I denied her pain, how I discarded her feelings and negated her. That's why I struggle to get over this moment and why even now, years later, it's still the single most painful memory I have of Leo's transition.

I can only imagine the courage it must have taken her to start to have that conversation with me. I found out later that she had, of course, been looking things up on the internet and had come across the term "transgender". She said it exactly described how she felt – trapped in the wrong body. Can you imagine how distressing that would be? We all have bits of our bodies we dislike or sometimes even hate, but can you imagine what it must be like for your whole body to just feel *wrong*? It's really hard to do.

Our GP explained it to me in a different way that helped me understand and put it in perspective by using my younger son, Luca, as an example. The GP said, "Think about if he started to grow breasts and have periods. You'd feel shocked, you'd want to help, and you'd immediately wonder what was wrong and what could you do about it. You'd be instantly full of hurt and worry, and you would understand that your son felt awful, betrayed by his body because it was malfunctioning in some horrible way. That's the experience of a transgender person." It makes you think, doesn't it? Straight away, it seems so clear and obvious. Of course there would be hurt, distress and worry. Of course that child would want to hide their body away. Of course they would feel saddened, worried and even embarrassed. And that was how my child felt, and I'd just brushed it all aside.

At the time, despite everything I've just said and how awful I still feel about that moment, I wasn't a complete monster. I was just a busy, harassed mum who wanted their child not to be upset – for her and for me. But I did at least notice the tears that accompanied that statement were more profuse and seemed somehow worse than a normal childhood worry. I sat on the bed beside E and tried to tuck her in. I said, more gently this time, how it was normal for someone of her age to start thinking more about her body and her identity. I said that teenage years and puberty, which she was fast approaching, were a time of massive change. I explained that often people wanted to try out different things – that they might be attracted to different people, and that was all okay and natural. But back then I knew absolutely nothing about gender identity, so I didn't realize that questioning and experimenting with gender could also be a part of this process. Therefore, I didn't include that in my little chat.

Around that time, Caitlyn Jenner had just come out as transgender, so her story was very in the spotlight. But I thought E was just confused about her sexuality and perhaps was gay. Or even just experimenting? I remembered feeling "boyish" when I was a kid, and I thought that it would be cooler to be a boy – they seemed to have more freedom than I did. Why couldn't I have just taken the time to listen instead of being cross and frustrated that it was bedtime? I still feel guilty and ashamed by my memories of this bedside chat. It was a pivotal moment for E telling me – she must have been building up to it for days and days, and I dismissed it with a few words. I let her down. I still feel so haunted by that conversation, and I still can't forgive myself for it.

* * *

Leo

I'm often asked when I realized I was trans and I always feel as if I'm giving a bit of a disappointing answer because, truthfully, I can never really recall. I don't remember specifically how I even found out what the word "transgender" was. It's important to note that around the time I came out, Caitlyn Jenner's transition was appearing in mainstream news, and there was heavy focus on the story, especially because she was a well-known public figure prior to her announcement that she intended to transition. Before her, I don't remember ever hearing about a transgender public figure or, in fact, anything about positive about transgender people prior to her story. It felt as though everyone knew there was such a thing, but it wasn't something to think or talk about. In films and TV shows, trans people seemed to me to be continuously misrepresented and included as a character of comic relief. It seemed and felt like trans people were a dirty little secret, something to gawk at and only speak about in whispers, something for everyone to share their opinion on.

Due to the lack of visibility of trans people in the UK at the time (though, of course, they existed), the kind of public discussions and debates on the topic of trans rights and issues did not exist as they do now. And discussions around safety and healthcare for trans people certainly didn't appear to be taken seriously. I think originally my parents believed that Caitlyn Jenner was where I "got the idea from", and that I was confused about my identity and sense of self, and therefore, perhaps subconsciously, projected those feelings onto her example to provide myself with an explanation. Of course, it later became apparent this wasn't the case. It frequently frustrates me that, for as long as I've been asked when I knew, I've always been unable to pinpoint it exactly, but I was certainly aware as a child that I felt different to other girls.

When I hit puberty – when I was 11 turning 12 – I started to notice that I was different and began to question myself and areas of my identity, though that wasn't quite how I thought about it then. I'd been having some trouble with my sexuality because at the time I had crushes on boys in school and I knew that was "normal" for girls to feel, but I was bewildered to realize that I was interested in girls too. I found this confusing because, even though it was roughly a decade ago, no one, let alone schoolchildren, seemed to talk about or understand the difference between gender and sexuality. Yet I knew there was more to it and that there was some other element of myself I couldn't grasp or reconcile. The fact that I was "a girl" was what I couldn't accept. So, I settled on thinking that I was just gay and tried to block out my attraction to boys because that felt like too much to cope with and understand, and that way I'd be making my feelings easier for others to accept. (This is something I think all queer people have done at some point, but, fellow queers, please tell me if I'm wrong.)

There was a particular day at school in Year 6, when the anxiety and stress that had been building for weeks – stemming from my confusion about myself and the feelings of discomfort I had surrounding being a girl, and being unable to understand why I was feeling the way I did – all came to a head. On this day, after getting upset in the classroom and not feeling comfortable talking to my teacher about it, I accepted her offer of visiting the school counsellor to discuss what was distressing me. After sitting in her room, crying quietly for a while, unable to decide how to phrase what I was feeling, the counsellor asked me what was wrong. I tried to explain how I felt, but I didn't have the vocabulary. Some things I told her that have stuck with me include, "I like girls. But as a boy," and, "I don't feel like I am a girl that likes girls. I only want to be with girls if I'm a boy." She looked at me as if I'd just told her,

"I think I'm an alien," yet she was still managing to be gentle and compassionate. I didn't expect her to understand or grasp what I had just told her because I couldn't make sense of it myself. That was the extent I was able to describe my feelings of displacement and distress without having the appropriate vocabulary and knowing what words like "trans" or "gender dysphoria" meant at the time. The frustration of not being able to make people understand how I felt was torturous, especially when it was causing me to feel so depressed and lost. All I needed was for someone to understand.

She asked whether I had explained to my parents what I had just told her. I said that I hadn't yet, but I wanted to. Not because I thought about transitioning – I had no idea that it was a possibility and something people did, or that it could ever be an option for me. It was because I have always had a close relationship with my parents, and I wanted them to know and acknowledge the way I was feeling, and how important what I was feeling was to me. I felt like I would be living a lie if I couldn't explain it to them. I didn't feel like their daughter, and I wanted them to understand, though I didn't really kid myself that they would. Sarah, the counsellor, asked if we should bring them in to talk it through with her, but I didn't want to do it there. I wanted to be in a space where I was more comfortable to have such an awkward and difficult conversation; plus, I didn't quite feel ready to do so. I spent the next few weeks mulling over our conversation and building up the courage to put everything into words.

Unfortunately, I think I knew deep down the reaction I was going to get, and I didn't expect that it would go well. Although my parents loved and respected me, I knew I was bound to be taken less seriously as a child coming out than if I was their 20-year-old telling them the same thing. Coming out as a transgender was such an uncommon thing to hear about or experience at that time. In fact, I never had the thought to google it or try to search for the words to tell them, despite the fact that the time we're discussing was only about ten years ago. As I've said before, the amount of media attention that trans issues and people get now has wildly increased, so it can seem unrealistic to say that I didn't know where to turn. Yet there was nowhere obvious to go to get support for having these conversations, or for parents who were experiencing it then, when we needed it.

When I told my mum, she didn't know what the word "transgender" was. She'd only heard of transsexuals, of transvestites, of drag ... which I think it's fair to say were the sorts of things and terms that came to mind for the average person if asked to picture "trans people" at that time. I knew it would look like I was being silly or that I'd made it up, but I just felt like I had to try my best to get them to listen and understand. I think that's why it took a few times of me explaining how I felt before they realized this was perhaps more serious than they first thought or would've liked it to have been. Before I first tried coming out to my mum, I tried to tell my dad.

It was night-time on a weekday. I thought I could only do it at night because I knew my parents were busy in the day and it never felt like there was an appropriate time to have the sort of discussion that I wanted to have with them. I also thought it was likely that I, or my parents, would get upset, so I decided the evening was the best time for it, so we could sleep it off, rather than ruminating for the rest of the day. I'd been in bed for a while, and had gone downstairs sobbing to my dad, who was by himself watching TV. Earlier that day, we were in the car, and there had been a piece on the radio that mentioned transgender people, most likely something about Caitlyn Jenner, though I don't recall exactly what was said. I'd asked him, "What do you think of those people?"

He answered, "Well, you know, it's their business." He obviously didn't know why I was asking and probably felt a bit uncomfortable discussing it, yet the question I knew I was asking him in that moment was, "What would you think if I said I was one of them?"

I don't remember my phrasing as well as I remember the conversation with my mum, but I'm sure it was very similar. I said,

"Do you remember what we were talking about earlier, in the car? I think I'm one of those people." He just kind of laughed and sort of scoffed – not in a horrible way, but as if I'd just told him a shit joke. It was clear he felt awkward and didn't have much to say and would probably rather I stopped talking about it and went back to sleep. He just said back, "You know, it's time to go to bed, Muppet. Come on, go back upstairs." And just like that, I had been shut down. I went back to my room and cried in my bed until I fell asleep. A couple of weeks later, I tried again with Mum.

Activity-wise, it was a normal day again – I'd gone to school, had dinner, got ready for bed. But I think if you've been upset by something before and you're having to face it again, you always feel much more emotional the second time round. I had been thinking about my conversation with my dad 24/7 for those past few weeks. I had been upset, crying in my room again as I had done multiple evenings before. I thought to myself, *I just have to stop.* I knew that if I could get it out into the open, and if I could get Mum and Dad to accept this was something I was truly experiencing, it would be the beginning of everyone coming to terms with it. And that's why I just tried to get it out of the way. I viewed it as a stepping stone, and I really needed to tell my parents – I just wanted them to understand. But I knew that because of how crazy it sounded to them, tonight wasn't going to be an instance of acceptance. I had been so worked up, and I don't know why I chose that evening exactly to talk to my mum, but I kept thinking, *I have to make a start.* I remember the exact words we said to each other as she was about to leave my room before I went to sleep.

"Mum, I think I'm a boy."

And Mum's reply, after a long pause, during which she was trying to rationalize and process what I had just told her, was:

"Oh E, don't be silly. *You're not a boy.*"

To a degree I expected my mum's reaction because I knew how out of the blue it would seem to her. I could understand how alien it would sound because it felt alien to me. I didn't expect her to give me a cuddle and tell me we could work this out. But it didn't make her response any easier to hear. When I was thinking about telling her, I don't think I thought in specific detail about what exactly she might say; I just predicted it would feel a bit like we weren't going to get anywhere right away, so I wasn't exactly wrong. But exactly what she said, the phrasing, *"You're not a boy"* – it felt like a slap in the face. My heart sunk.

When this is how you've felt and recognized yourself your whole life, and you finally understand this is the part of you that has made you feel so different for all these years, having to hear such a stark and striking lack of acceptance and empathy from your parent … it's difficult to know what to liken it to. I suppose it felt as if I had said to her, "This is the most important thing in the world to me, and if I can never live and be accepted by you as your son, I don't know if I'll ever be truly happy." And to be met with her response felt as if she'd told me that it was categorically never going to happen. Of course, I don't blame my mum for what she said because she didn't understand at the time how strongly I felt and how desperate I was in that moment for her approval because I couldn't articulate it to her. There was no way I could make her realize what it felt like being me or why her acceptance was so important. All I think she saw was her young, impressionable – and at the time, hysterical – child who was up too late and had got worked up over something silly and ridiculous.

After I'd had my first attempts to talk to my parents, the next conversation I had about it was a week or so later. I was with my best friend at the time, Tiffany, and her mum, at a park in our area. Tiffany was probably the only person at the time that knew how I felt and accepted me in the same way as she had before. All she knew was that I was her friend and I was struggling. I told her about when I'd tried to speak to my parents and how disheartened and upset those conversations had made me, and she was incredibly supportive. Whilst we were talking about it, naturally, I got upset and explained to her, "I just don't know what to do. I just want my parents to understand. I'm not saying we need to go anywhere with it soon, I just want them to know how I feel and to be able to sympathize, at least. I wish that just for one day, they could experience what it was like be in my body and feel how I feel because I know then they would get it." Tiffany's mum came over, concerned after seeing me get so upset, and asked me what was wrong. Tiffany and I tried our best to explain it to her. She was amazing, but it can't be overlooked that it's much easier to be sympathetic and understanding in a situation that you aren't experiencing and struggling with personally. She suggested, "Why don't I try and have a chat with your mum, and when I drop you off, just say you've been upset today, and this is why. Do you want me to do that? Would that be okay?" And I agreed because I think I might have known that hearing from another parent how upset I'd been might demonstrate to my mum that I wanted my feelings to be recognized and taken seriously. I thought that having to have that awkward conversation with my friend's mum might make it sink in that this was something that was distressing me, and that we needed to have more of a talk about it.

I remember when my mum and Tiffany's mum were talking at the door. I'd gone into the kitchen but was quite unsuccessfully attempting to eavesdrop on the conversation. I wanted to know what my mum would say about it, to know what her response would be. Tiffany's mum said I was really upset that day. She explained what I'd been saying about how I felt. But I couldn't really hear what was being said.

When Mum came back in, she wore a concerned look on her face. I could tell she felt slightly embarrassed, but also confused and anxious. We had a chat at the kitchen table about what I had said to Tiffany and her mum, both getting quite teary, and after a while, she suggested, "Why don't we go to the GP and see what they have to say? Maybe they could be of some help?" And in that moment, for the first time in months, I felt a glimmer of hope.

Chapter 2

GROWING UP

Gemma

I was pretty sure I didn't want children for most of my early adult life. In fact, I was still pretty sure there was a way I could find out how to be a Jedi and do that instead. (I'm still looking.) I left home when I was 17 to live with my first "proper" boyfriend and thought myself very grown up, although we lived mainly on chips. By the time I was 19, we'd split up, I'd moved back home and managed to get back together with my childhood school sweetheart, and we were dating again. Within a year we were living together in Nottingham and got married when I was just 21. It seems so early to be married at that age now, but my parents had been the same age when they married, and so were most other people's parents, too. I married Kev on the basis that neither of us wanted children, or if we did, it was in some unforeseeable future. By the time I was 27, a lot had happened, most of which involved two people who got married very young growing up and, as often happens, had grown apart. I remember having a dinner party for my 27th birthday, being bored and thinking my life – and any fun in it – was over. You won't be surprised to learn that we split up not long afterwards.

At that point I decided it was too late to have children anyway and thought very seriously about being sterilized so that I would never have to worry about it again. I remember talking to my mum and she counselled against it. Although they had had me very young (my parents were only 20 when I came along), and my dad had been sterilized at 24, Mum said there was always a possibility things might change and not to close any doors just yet. Hindsight really is a wonderful thing.

Aged 28 and living on my own in a flat in Bedford, I met Bill. He came to give me a quote for decorating my hallway ceiling, which he was very amused to discover had taken me an entire day, three trips to the local DIY store and three lots of brushes and rollers to paint badly. It wasn't love at first sight as much as it was lust, to be honest, but that's not a bad start to a relationship when you're both grown up and single. I wasn't looking for anything serious, but it soon became that way, and we got married a few days after I turned 30. We'd both been married before, so rather than a big church do, we went to Fiji to get married on our own and have our honeymoon at the same time.

Bill was already a dad to two (then) small boys, aged three and six. He didn't have a great relationship with their mum at that point, sadly, so he only got to see them at weekends. I never really felt like their stepmum back then and was sad I didn't have a chance to get closer to them, but it's just how it was. However, it was clear that Bill loved being a dad. He said it was always something he'd wanted to be, so he'd had his children young. After we were married, I started to change my mind about parenthood, and pretty soon, it was me who broached the subject with him. We had married assuming we wouldn't have kids, and as Bill already had his boys, neither of us thought that would change. But life has a funny way of making you rethink things, and so we quite soon decided we would try and have a family of our own. It didn't take long – I fell pregnant the first month we tried! (Not the same story with my second pregnancy, which took us over a year of trying.)

I am lucky in that I haven't had to spend much time in hospitals, which is just as well because I'm really not good with them – or with blood, injections or anything else, really. When I was pregnant with

E, I was told I needed to have a blood test, so off I went to get it. But I almost passed out. I was literally shaking with fear beforehand and crying. When I left the room where they eventually managed to get enough blood for the relevant tests, I was in an absolute state. I remember thinking as I was ushered past the waiting queue by my husband, still shaking and snotting everywhere, that people sitting in the waiting room and watching me go past must have thought I'd been told some kind of awful news. So, hospitals and I didn't make for a great mix.

Five months in, we went back to hospital for our first scan. The writing on the scan was "(??)", which meant they couldn't be sure what the sex of our baby was, but they thought it might be a girl, as there didn't seem to be any obvious male genitalia. I remember, the piece of paper said "Girl?". Seems ironic in hindsight that, even then, there was a question about our child's gender. Looking back now, it was the first time that it really hit home to me that genitals = sex of the baby. A defining feature in whether they are there or not there ... all down to whether there was a willy in the picture. It wasn't until our next scan much later that it was confirmed as likely (still not definite!) that we were having a girl, and I remember spending a lot of time thinking about what that might mean.

Much later, in family counselling, one of our counsellors, Phil, said that part of what we needed to do in our situation was think about the stories we had built up around our daughter and what life might be like with her, and start to let those go. Well, from my pregnancy onward, I started building up my stories, I guess. I was delighted to have a girl. I'm sure I would have been equally delighted to have a boy. It's one of those weird things, isn't it ... whatever your first baby is, you're just pleased to have a child that's well, healthy and happy. I knew what I'd looked like as a little girl and assumed she'd look kind of like me. I didn't go out and buy lots of girly clothes. She was never going to be decked out in pink, frills and bows. But it is surprising how much of yourself you project onto your unborn children. I bought lots of colourful clothes – which were closer to unisex than anything else – toys and books. My kids were always going to have lots of books. Books and stories were a massive part of my upbringing, from bedtime stories to stories of magic, fairies and heroes from my grandma (and even manuscripts of stories from her mum!), to teenage escapism. My love of *The Hobbit* was born then, and I have continued to read it and a plethora of other books every year since I was old enough to get through it.

Honestly, I don't think I was a great mum initially. I'd taken the approach to motherhood that I took to everything else – read everything I could, go to the classes to learn how to do it properly, worry a lot and try to plan everything. I felt a bit reassured that Bill already had kids – I thought at least I'd have an experienced pair of hands around. My mum and dad lived in Spain, though. I didn't have friends with kids that lived close to me. And I wasn't particularly close to my mother-in-law, who is considerably older than my mum and dad. So, Bill was really it in terms of support. In the run up to the birth, I had a few scares, which were pretty "normal" things. My blood pressure went quite high, and I had to spend a night in hospital having it monitored. I'd put on loads of weight and felt terrible. My oedema was so bad I used to press my fingers into my shins like they were made of jelly and see the indents they left behind. But all in all, I was lucky with my pregnancy. I wasn't too sick. I think I only actually threw up twice, although I did feel nauseous quite a lot. I thought I'd got off lightly.

Time passed, I got bigger and bigger, and the due date came and went. In the meantime, we'd got boys names that we agreed on straight away. We hadn't decided on a girl's name, but E, Rosa and Lola were all in the running. We decided to see what she looked like when she came out. That moment would come eventually – after two weeks and another blood pressure scare, the decision was made to induce me.

After a relatively easy pregnancy, giving birth was another matter. I was quite late but thought if I got any bigger, I might actually explode! I'd carefully planned a home birth with a birthing pool and had got it all booked. I really hate hospitals, and when my antenatal class took a tour of the maternity suite, I was done for. I was crying on the way round and thinking that I couldn't possibly see myself giving birth in hospital. I had a weird kind of terror for hospitals, perhaps not helped by my only real experience of them being when my grandma, and then later my grandad, died in hospital, and my own experience of being admitted to A&E after a serious car crash with my boyfriend when I was 16.

Grandma, who died of lung cancer, was moved to a small side room in Addenbrookes, and as a family we waited with her, watching her withering away, losing her consciousness and being dehumanized until she passed. It was the first time I'd ever seen a dead body, and I couldn't believe that the crumpled, empty husk on the bed used to be my grandma. My grandad was admitted as an emergency years later after a heart attack. Again, I saw him in intensive care, wired up to machines that were breathing for him while his organs failed. I remember whispering to him that we would look after Nanna (Grandma was my mum's mum. Grandad was my dad's dad). He looked like a wax figure, and it was heart-breaking because although he hadn't wasted away like Grandma, he looked grey and unreal. We were told by the doctor that there was no hope for Grandad as his systems were shutting down, so they would give us some time to think and be on our own, and then if we agreed, they would turn off the life support machine at 8pm. At 7:55pm, the doctor came in to tell us that Grandad had just died. I still think he was trying to save us from making a terrible decision.

So, my experience of hospitals was traumatic, to say the least.

When I started to experience problems with my blood pressure, I was told that the home birth I'd wanted was no longer an option, and the doctors kept a closer eye on me. So, when the decision was taken to induce me, I was terrified. This was the very opposite of what I'd hoped for, and even worse, I was being taken into hospital to have my baby forced out of me – at least that's what it felt like.

I was admitted after lunch and taken to a room where I would start my labour. At the very best of times, I hate needles, and of course, the first thing I needed was a needle inserted into the back of my hand to give me the drugs that would start my labour. (Actually, that was the second thing. The first thing was an inspection of my cervix – the first of many, but the most excruciatingly embarrassing one because at that point, before you actually give birth, you still care).

It was decided to break my waters manually, so off we went. This involved a device that looked a bit like a hook that my nanna used to use in her knitting, being inserted and scraped over the baby's head in an attempt to break the bag of amniotic fluid surrounding her, but even that didn't go according to plan. (When E did eventually emerge, she had huge red scratches on top of her head from the attempts.) I was given some gas and air to help me through the process, which dulled the pain but also made me feel like I was drunk, with a spinning head and spinning room around me. Not pleasant at all!

It only went downhill from there. I know at the NCT class they told me the only thing to expect at a first-time birth was that nothing could be expected. After the first hour, the nurse came back to check me and check the baby, and nothing much was happening. Contractions were weak and too far apart, and when they checked my cervix again (still agonizingly embarrassing) – no dice. So, the drugs dial was turned up in the hope that contractions would get going properly. They did. That was not much fun, and pretty soon, I vomited the piece of chocolate cake I'd eaten earlier that morning. (Don't judge me, I was fed up and very pregnant!) After another couple of hours and some stronger contractions, the pain became harder to manage, and gas and air, which had seemed like fun earlier, stopped having much of an effect. The doctor then came in to give me an epidural. By the looks of it, it was a good job I couldn't see what was going on, as Bill's face went pale when he saw the needle. The doctor had me sit on the edge of the bed while he put the epidural in. I was literally shivering like a cold dog at the time. He was trying to tell me to take deep breaths and relax, but I was scared shitless. My whole body would shake, freeze and then start again. I can understand why that made putting a huge needle into my spine difficult, and maybe that was why, in turn, the epidural didn't really work very well.

I was told to stay in bed and I was on my back. The contractions were horrible, and the epidural wasn't really blocking out the pain, especially on one side. I remember bunching up on one side of the bed when the waves of pain crashed over me, and then trying to push away from the bottom of the bed with my arms braced on the side rails. It wasn't just me in distress – the baby's heartbeat seemed to be going a bit wrong, and the doctors were becoming more concerned about her. Then, the team noticed that the baby had passed some meconium, which is a warning of distress in an unborn baby, and they started to worry about getting her out. More and more people began crowding into the room. On one contraction, I'm fairly sure I did a poo myself, and thank God, someone just cleared me up and carried on. Absolutely mortifying. I now had my legs in stirrups so more and more people could look up my insides. At one point between contractions, I counted 14 people in the room – I mean, what the hell? I guess with hindsight they were probably getting ready to do an emergency caesarean, as the baby was in some distress. So was I. I've never felt so scared, so out of control and in so much pain before or since. No wonder no one tells you what childbirth can really be like – you'd never do it! I'd seen it on the TV, of course … I knew there was some pain and some sweating … but I didn't realize it could go on for so long and be so many different types of awful. Complete and utter lack of dignity and privacy. Almost total disregard for what I was feeling or going through apart from how much pain I was in. (I understand that the priority in these situations is the baby, but surely if I was at least less terrified, that would have been better for the baby, too?) Pain like I couldn't believe. And fear. A lot of fear. It went on for a bizarre amount of time that seemed like (and was) hours, and yet all blurred together in one horrible, stretched-out nightmare moment. A ventouse was used – a weird vacuum-like machine attached to the baby's head, which literally, finally, pulled her out of me.

The pain was so bad, I was just screaming and screaming. I was lost in it and overwhelmed by it. I remember the midwife trying to talk to me. I can't remember anything about her – what she looked like, how old she was … all I remember is her making me look her in the eyes. She said, "Gemma, pay attention to me. You're losing it." I thought she meant I was losing the baby. At that moment, I didn't care if I did. The pain was so bad, I just wanted it to stop – at any cost. Much later I realized she was trying to get me to focus and be in the world, not lost in my pain. But man, those were not the right words to say to me at that point.

I remember a single moment of fire-like pain between my legs, and then a weird relief. It was my body literally tearing apart to let my baby out. Blood gushed onto the sheets, which were whipped away, and the head finally emerged, with the rest of the baby not too far behind. Then, there she was – quickly wrapped in a towel and plonked on me. Her head was, of course, all bent out of shape and cone-like from where the ventouse machine had tugged her, and her scalp was covered in red stripes from the knitting-needle hook. Poor baby girl. What a way to come into the world.

The only upside was being presented with my daughter at the end of it, still feeling battered, sick, bleeding and out of it. It was the first time I'd seen Bill cry. He told me he'd always wanted a girl. Her nightmare might have been over – but mine wasn't. We had some time to get to know each other a bit, say hello and for Bill to hold her. But after a few minutes, the team started getting ready for the placenta to come out. Except it didn't. And didn't. And didn't.

I received another injection and a few other things that were meant to help. Still nothing. I had torn badly, so the decision was made to take me into surgery, to get me stitched up and manually remove the placenta. So, Bill took E off to a room, and I was left in a corridor for a bit – I have no idea how long I was there, but it felt sad and lonely. I was bereft.

When I was wheeled into surgery, things didn't improve. I was still conscious but felt basically like I was completely drunk. I felt sick and out of control, and had no real idea what was going on. Again, I remember the feeling of shame and indignity of someone having their arm inside me almost up to the elbow – the blood lines on the gloves made me feel sick, they were so far up. I could also feel pain right inside me … it felt unnatural and wrong that I should be aware of something inside my body like that. I remember that two nurses were talking to each other about everyday stuff over me, like I was a corpse. And I felt halfway to being one. A particularly horrible moment was when one of them had to put a painkiller up my bum. One nurse gave the tablet to the other one, who said, "I get all the best jobs." I didn't feel it go in, but I did die a bit inside. Even typing this now is making me feel sad and hopeless – the whole experience was just fucking awful. I was stitched up, inside and out, and wheeled back to a recovery room. By that time, I felt pretty much subhuman, sweaty, bloody, exhausted, tearful – the whole works.

The first couple of hours after the birth, I was semi-conscious in an operating theatre, and then I was semi-conscious and very lonely in a room somewhere recovering. The birth already seemed hours away. I was eventually wheeled into a room and reunited with Bill and E, where I was allowed to see them briefly before Bill went home, exhausted, and E and I went to the ward, exhausted too. I was lucky enough (or damaged enough?!) to have a private room, and E was wheeled in beside me.

She was so tiny and so dependent, and I had no real idea what to do. I held her, of course, and tried to reconcile the fact that she used to be in me and now was in my arms. It was the weirdest-ever feeling – completely surreal. I mainly felt totally unprepared. Any movement or squeak and I wasn't sure what to do. I still couldn't really move very well but remember lifting her out (or perhaps she was handed to me, it's a bit of a blur) and trying to feed her. I'd really, really wanted to breastfeed. I knew how important it was for the baby. I knew how much she needed the nourishment and the good bugs I could pass on to her. I knew it would help me lose the baby weight. I really wanted to be able to do it so badly. I was heartbroken all over again when I couldn't get it to work. My milk just wouldn't come. A midwife tried to help me. E tried to latch on, but nothing worked. I was just exhausted and tearful, and I couldn't believe I was denied the joy of feeding my baby, which I felt like I deserved at the end of my birth experience. I was deemed too exhausted to look after her, so the midwife took her to the nursery to get her looked after and said they would bring her back in the morning. I was exhausted and sore and didn't need much persuading. I cried myself to sleep.

So, my introduction to parenthood was pretty brutal, and it didn't get easier! For some reason, I couldn't breastfeed. The next morning, E was brought back to me, and we tried again. And again. A midwife tried to help. A breastfeeding specialist tried to help. Just about everyone who walked in the room tried to help. Eventually, a few drops of milk started to come out, but only after agonizing minutes passed of us trying, E crying, me crying and resting and trying again. The breastfeeding specialist recommended I get a breast pump, so at least E could have my milk, and she gave me one to try. For those first few days, my baby was fed formula while I tried to recover. I was moved to a ward and catheterized because I couldn't wee. Of course, that gave me a urine infection. Basically, I was shot to pieces. I felt like I had failed miserably as a new mother. I tried and tried – with midwives, with home visits. I tried at every feed. But for some reason, my milk didn't come in fast enough, E got frustrated, I got tense, and it just didn't happen.

Coming home felt like not just an anticlimax, but also a realization. The exhaustion wasn't going away ... it wasn't getting a chance to. Anyone who has been a parent knows what the next few weeks are like – exhausting, confusing, with the washing machine on constantly! I was struggling physically and ended up seeing a counsellor to talk about the birth, as I kept getting flashbacks and couldn't seem to get over it. I think my unpreparedness, coupled with the trauma of it, just seemed to make it worse. I also felt terrible guilt because at the point I thought the midwife had told me I was losing the baby and the pain was so bad, I didn't care and just wanted it to stop. I couldn't get over the fact I felt like I'd put myself first.

Clearly, becoming a new mum was a real learning process, one not helped by the fact that between us, we still couldn't seem to work out breastfeeding. I really wanted to, but I couldn't seem to relax enough to let the milk flow, and I got upset when E couldn't latch on. We tried and tried, and I ended up getting more and more upset. So, in the end, I expressed – or pumped – all E's milk for the first three months. I'd express and then give it to her in a bottle, so feeding took twice as long every time. She was also a terrible sleeper. I'd spend hours with her, feeding her, shushing her, cuddling her, but every single time I gently put her down in her bed, she'd wake up. And cry. Getting her to sleep took hours, and then she woke up again so quickly. In the first few weeks, she was waking up four or five times a night. Bill didn't wake up, but I always did. I always went to her. I started to resent the fact that Bill could sleep through the crying ... but also, just that he could sleep at all! On nights when E really wouldn't settle and I was getting to the end of my tether, I would wake Bill. It was only rarely and only when I'd already been awake for hours. He would take E, and I guess because he was so much calmer than me, she would settle and finally sleep.

Looking back now, I'm sure so much of this was because of my sense of failure, worry and tension about everything. I couldn't possibly relax, so how could she? Again, parents anywhere will recognize this story I'm sure, but my God ... we've all been through it. Why the hell don't we all do more to support new parents?

Despite all these problems and my constant exhaustion, I was absolutely overwhelmed by the love I felt for E. I never wanted to put her down. I thought she was incredible, this tiny human being who was all mine (well, and Bill's but mainly mine!). She was so dependent on me for everything, and I wanted to give her everything she needed. I didn't even like giving her to other people to hold. Nicknamed "Froggy legs" because she was so skinny (only about 6lbs when she was born, and she lost a bit of weight initially because of our feeding problems), I was besotted. Bill was amazing with her too, and we tried to start getting on with a "normal" life. I would walk her in her pram and be so happy to be with her. We were lucky that although I was the main breadwinner, I was able to work quite a lot from home, and Bill could fit his work in around us both, so he became the main carer. For the first year, E stayed at home with Bill, and we were both around a lot for her, which I realize put us in a very different position to most new parents. She was still a terrible sleeper, but somehow, I managed to adjust to being woken two or three times a night and could sleep in when Bill woke up with her for the early feed. Our life with a daughter was underway.

As E started to grow up, despite the fact she was still a terrible sleeper, she was a good-natured, happy little girl. She went to nursery when she was about one, and quickly made friends and especially loved one of the girls who looked after her. Of course, in those early years, E wore whatever clothes we put her in. I've never been a huge fan of girly clothes and princess outfits – nothing against those kids and parents who love them, I just didn't, and E didn't seem bothered either. She was always happiest in trousers and a hoodie, and that's pretty much what she lived in. When she was about three or four and started to realize there was a difference between girls and boys, she decided that she was a boy. "I'm a boy and I want to be called John Lewis" is what she told us. Even today, we chuckle at that. We didn't think anything of it and laughed it off. Now I know that trans kids often express these types of thoughts and feelings when they're this young. To me it makes sense ... as soon as they realize there are boys and girls, they start to think about whether they "fit" into the gender they're supposed to be – and in E's case, she thought she didn't.

Certainly as she got older, she became more "boyish", but again, we didn't see any issue with that or think anything of it. She was always really pleased if we went into a shop and someone mistook her for a boy. I did notice how differently people treated her if she was seen as a boy too ... more of an "all right, mate?" and comments about which football team she liked, or questions about if she was "running us ragged" or stuff like that. It occurred to me that these weren't questions that a stranger would ask about a girl. It was then that the subtleties of how we bring up kids and just how gendered it is started to show a bit for me.

E went through phases of being more and then less "girly" in her dress and appearance. I remember one year at primary school, she wanted to go back to school in a dress and made me buy one before the beginning of term, as she'd previously only ever worn trousers. She looked pretty in the little yellow gingham dress that was the school's summer uniform option for girls, but it lasted less than a week. Then when she was about eight, we decided she was old enough to come along to a special dinner I was having to celebrate my 40th birthday. She wore a gorgeous dress and cardigan and sparkly red shoes. After the main course, completely unprompted, she stood up and proposed a toast! I have no idea how she knew what to do, as it was the first time she'd been out with us in the evening, and it's not as if we go to places where people propose toasts! But I was so proud of her and her maturity. I had tears shining in my eyes as I said to Bill, "Our little girl is growing up." I think that was the last time I remember seeing her in a dress.

My best friend, Teresa, was a fitness instructor and taught dance classes. E came along with me to some Body Jam classes. I was completely hopeless, but E was pretty good, and Teresa had some contacts in Bedford who taught street dance. She introduced us to Rio, who danced in a proper crew and taught kids of all ages how to street dance. We went along to a class in town, and E was super shy (very unlike her). We had to bribe her with a can of Coke and a fiver to even get her to try it (I know, I know, another black mark in the parenting book for me). For the first class, she basically stood on the sidelines and wouldn't join in at all. But she did go back for another class. And another one. And then we discovered not only that she liked it, but she was really good at it! The guys who made up the Apex crew – Rio, Sam, Eli and JMC – were absolute stars and so cool. They were great kids who were all amazing dancers, and all brilliant with the kids they taught. It was so fantastic seeing all these little dancers who looked up to them, wanted to be them and loved hanging out with them. It really was a big family, and a great thing for the kids to be involved with.

Street dance became a big part of E's life, with classes every week and regular competitions with the crew and as a solo dancer at the same events. Quite a few weekends turned into spending the day in a sports hall surrounded by kids and loud dance and hip-hop music. But it was great fun, and I met my friend Jo, another dance mum, through the group, and we're still mates a decade later.

Of course, as a street dancer, E was really hiding in plain sight. All the kids wore baseball caps, hoodies and baggy trousers, so it was natural that she would too. A few of the girls who attended classes were more "girly", wearing long hair and cropped tops, but E was good at the stuff that more boys were good at – the popping and locking and body isolations that made her a "popper". Members of the crew all got nicknames for when they competed, and E's was "Star Popper". She was talented and started to do well in competitions on her own and as part of the young Apex crew. She especially loved it when there were solo dance-offs, as she was almost always dancing with, and against, boys, and was always "mistaken" for a boy. She continued to do well, and at one competition, she qualified to dance at The O2 arena in London for a chance to represent the UK in the European Hip-Hop Championships.

We went along to The O2, and Rio and a few other crew members came with us too. It was nerve-wracking, and that was just as an audience member! We jammed into our seats in a small, dark room and watched a procession of youngsters come onto the stage in nervous batches. Then, the music would bang out, and they would start moving. We watched a bunch of rounds, and then it was E's turn in the under-12s "Electric Boogie" category (what a name!). She came onto the stage with a small group of other kids, the music started, and they were underway! The audition literally only lasted a couple of minutes, and because you didn't know which piece of music you were going to get, you couldn't really prepare. Also, one of the skills of street dance was being able to move according to the music – showing off your musicality and inventiveness by linking your moves to the music. When the results came in, she got through! It was such an amazing moment, and we were so proud! I was crying (obviously), Bill was crying, and even Rio was crying. It was a real high. She qualified as part of the team and was selected to represent the UK in her category in the European Championships in Slovenia, where she went on to win a bronze medal.

So, street dance was a huge part of E's childhood and certainly helped in her self-development and in building her confidence. The strong link to boys' clothes also helped in giving her a chance to present herself in a way she felt more comfortable with, too. It was not too long after this period that E came out, and unfortunately that coincided with the crew disintegrating, with some of the senior members moving away and Rio eventually going to live abroad. It's a great shame that they weren't still around during the period of E coming out, as I feel like the community would have been supportive and given E some stability in her life at a time when she desperately needed it.

There were a couple of other experiences from E's childhood that I want to share because, unlike the positivity that came with street dance, they are hard and personal, and I want other parents who might be in the same position to know that you can get through them, despite making horrible mistakes at the time.

One is about going swimming. Ever since she was small, I took E swimming, and the same with Luca when he came along. It's a fun thing to do when your kids are small, but it's also an important skill, and for me, for some reason (and I have absolutely no idea where this came from!), I was always worried about them drowning. My mum and dad lived in Menorca, a beautiful island, where the capital, Mahon, sits right on a deep harbour. Whenever we used to go for coffee or food by the harbour, which was often, especially when the kids were small and we needed a cheap holiday destination, I would have this horrible underlying fear that the kids would somehow manage to fall in the water. Bizarre.

Anyway, E was a good swimmer. When Luca was a bit older, we took them both for lessons. E was a natural, and with her long, skinny frame, she cut through the water once she learnt how to breathe properly, and her teacher said she had great promise. So swimming was something that I took the kids to do regularly. (Bill can't really swim, and even on all those holidays in Menorca, he rarely even got into the pool, except on the odd occasion to play with the kids when we all bullied him into it!)

But as E started to become more and more unhappy with her female body, she became less keen on swimming. It was a shame, as it was a good way of doing something with both the kids, and where they would be happy playing with each other too, which allowed me to swim a few lengths in between games. One day, we were getting ready to go swimming. Normally, the kids would put their swimwear on under their clothes to minimize the time it took to get into the water once we arrived at the pool. E was in the downstairs bathroom getting changed but didn't want to put her costume on. Again, I was in "get things done" mode and chivvied her to hurry up. We (I) wanted to get to the pool early before it got too busy, and time was ticking away. I started to get impatient (I know, again ... you'd think I'd learn, but I just don't), and E started to get upset. I went into the bathroom where she was and could see she hadn't got changed. I left the door open, as Luca was in the hallway and the bathroom was quite big, as it had been made to accommodate a wheelchair. I thrust the swimsuit at E, who was just standing there.

"Come on, E, we need to go. Get changed now!"

She answered, "No, I don't want to."

"What do you mean, you don't want to? We've been talking about going swimming all morning, come on ..."

"I don't want to wear that costume. I don't want people to see me."

"Oh, don't be silly. If we go now, no one will even be there!"

"No, I don't want to wear that."

"Oh, for God's sake – of course you have to wear that. What else can you wear to go swimming?"

"I don't want to. I don't want to go."

I could see tears welling up in E's eyes. I could feel the internal heat of my frustration, not just with the situation and trying to get out of the house, but that again, I hadn't handled things well. Instead of facing up to this, I'm ashamed to say that I had no patience at all. There was my child, crying, feeling sad and uncomfortable about her body, and once again, I showed absolutely zero empathy. Instead, I just got cross that we were wasting time, that she was being "silly". *Argh* ... horrible. Again, I just feel ashamed by my behaviour looking at back at it. Even worse, I just left and took Luca swimming without her, leaving Bill to pick up the pieces. She was in tears, and I just said to Bill, "She doesn't want to come. So, I'm just going to take Luca." With that, I took Luca out to the car and left. Shit, Leo ... I'm sorry (again). Safe to say, that was the last time I took E swimming – or that she wanted to go – for a long, long time.

At that time, Luca would have been about seven, and as I strapped him into his child seat, I was frustrated and upset. I could feel tears in my own eyes, as I just hate seeing my kids upset – even if I'm the cause. Obviously, Luca wanted to know why E wasn't coming swimming with us. Swimming with his sister was way more fun than swimming with his mum. It was the first time I remember trying to explain a bit to Luca about what was going on. I said to him, "You know how you know you're a boy? And E is a girl? Well, sometimes people don't always feel like a girl or a boy, even though they might seem like one. E has told us that she doesn't feel like a girl, but that she feels like a boy. And so, some things are feeling harder for her. I think wearing a swimsuit, instead of trunks like you, is making her feel bad, so she doesn't want to wear one. So, she's decided she doesn't want to go swimming today." Of course, seven-year-old Luca seemed pretty unfazed by the whole thing and just said, "Will she go swimming another day?" to which the only answer seemed to be, "I should think so." Poor Luca – I don't think I was much fun in the pool that day with him, and I felt like a black cloud was hanging over me for the rest of the day, too.

Half-a-dozen years later, Leo would very occasionally go swimming with a rash vest on, only on holiday and only in my mum and dad's pool, never in public. Thankfully, since his surgery, he has been swimming more and will occasionally swim in public, though he gets worried people will notice his scars and somehow realize he's trans. I think his scars are quite hard to see, as they have faded a lot and he has quite a lot of chest hair now. But I guess if you know what to look for, they are pretty clearly the scars of a double mastectomy, and there's only one reason a young guy in his early 20s would have them.

For me, the other notable (for being awful) moment was when E started her menstrual cycle. We had known it was coming, of course, just because of her age and because she had started to develop some breast tissue. I wanted to do something to help her feel better. I wanted her to see that this was the start of her journey into being a woman. I hoped that her thoughts of being a boy would start to pass as she grew up and felt more feminine. (When I did some research online, it seemed to suggest that most kids who "thought" they were transgender would change their mind when they hit puberty. God knows where I read that, and of course it's absolute tripe – I hope that now there is better information out there than that, at least!) All that puberty showed us was how much E *was* transgender – I saw a happy, well-balanced young girl turned into a sad, inward-looking and despairing child. So, what could I do to help? Sit down and talk to her about how she was feeling? Try to understand how she felt "betrayed by [her] body" (those are the precise words Leo used to describe it later)? Not miss another chance to be sympathetic? Learn from my past mistakes on these big conversations? No, of course not. I fucked up – again. Because, of course, I didn't really want her to go down this path to transition. I was terrified of what it would mean for her – misery, pain, being "different", having to struggle throughout her life, having difficulty finding love … basically everything. I was catastrophizing in a big way. I just wanted it all to go away and make it all better. What makes everything better? Presents, I thought to myself. I proudly walked into E's bedroom after she'd been crying, carrying my old MacBook. I gave it to E, saying, "I just want you to realize that there are some upsides to being a girl." I wanted to acknowledge that she was growing up and thought a "grown-up" present would help.

For fuck's sake. Do you hate me? I hate me.

* * *

A NOTE ABOUT TOMBOYS – GEMMA

"Tomboys" is a term I see bandied around a lot on social media when it comes to trans kids, especially FTM (female-to-male, like Leo) trans kids. Most often, I've seen it in the comments of posts – "I was a tomboy, but I grew out of it" seems to be the most common response to FTM stories. I have seen it once or twice where people have assumed that a trans kid is just a tomboy "gone wrong", or one that's been too indulged, or someone who's habits have been "taken too far". Those statements are usually followed by some kind of comment like, "Thank God that back in my day, you could just be a tomboy." It does honestly feel like sometimes people think there's this big, hairy trans monster machine that goes around looking for tomboys, greedily sucks them up and spits out trans boys.

I do understand the confusion – I think. When I was ten or thereabouts, I went through a distinctly tomboy-ish stage, by which I mean I stopped with the fascination for frilly dresses, wore mainly jeans or cords (usually horribly mismatched with clashing prints ... it was the '70s!) and was also generally covered in dirt. I know everyone looks fondly back at their childhood, but I was pretty lucky in mine. I grew up in a small village, which was rural and felt safe. When I was very young, I used to play in the road – literally. (My dad tells a story about how, when I was about five, I took my little wicker chair and sat in the middle of the road. My dog came to sit with me.)

Anyway, back to being a tomboy. I played out. By "playing out", what I mean is, I told my mum I was going out with my friends, and then we met up somewhere in the village and played in the ditches and fields. We built castles out of haybales in the summer and started campfires in the ditches behind the vicarage. I was not a troublemaker, despite what that might sound like, but I was a kid. A normal kid. Some people called me a tomboy. I had short hair and wore clothes that meant I could easily be mistaken for a boy. I liked playing out with my friends – boys and girls – and I was pretty happy.

But, and it's a pretty massive "but" in the tomboy debate – I DID NOT *FEEL* LIKE A BOY. I thought that boys sometimes had it easier because it seemed like they were allowed to play out more and were sort of expected to come home dirty, while some of my friends who were girls were not. So, I was a bit jealous of them. Also, I thought they often had clothes that were cooler. Even at that age, I was aware of a kind of pressure that meant girls were expected to be cleaner (why *is* that?!), behave more nicely, be kinder to others and look after people more than boys. So sure, I was a tomboy. But also, wasn't I just a kid who was allowed to dress myself and so I wore what was comfortable for playing out? And hung around with boys doing boy stuff just because it was cool? At that point, I didn't see any of this as a response to gender per se, but of course, it was all gender based. These expectations of what a girl should do/say/look like, compared to what a boy should do/say/look like, meant that, to ten-year-old me, behaving like a boy was more fun. But again ... that didn't mean I felt like a boy or wanted to somehow be a boy. So, when people criticize Leo, or any other trans boys, by saying they were a tomboy but "thank God" no one allowed them to "take it too far" (i.e., the hairy trans machine didn't suck them up and spit them out as a trans boy), that's because, dare I say it, they also didn't FEEL like a boy, didn't SAY they were a boy, didn't CRY AT NIGHT because they weren't a boy, didn't feel a MASSIVE sense of wrong-ness in their body because they weren't a boy. See what I mean? Being a tomboy does not equal being a trans boy. They *might* look externally similar, I guess. But one is just a girl doing stuff that we now recognize were labelled as "boy" behaviours, one IS A BOY. Blimey ... I hope that makes sense.

So, unsurprisingly, when Leo was little, we also called him a tomboy. Because that's the language Bill and I grew up with and what people understood. Here was a girl, dressing like a boy, behaving like a boy, looking like a boy. Easy … a tomboy! I'm not sure if trans kids now have it easier or harder when they behave and look like the gender that is not the one they were assigned at birth. There definitely seems to be a real anxiety, usually from people who don't understand much about trans issues (in my experience, anyway), that tomboys will morph into trans kids, and I don't really get where that comes from. Even worse, some people seem to think that exhibiting any sort of non-cis-identifying behaviour (non-cis is short for non-cisgender, meaning a person doesn't identify with the sex they were assigned at birth) will mean that a well-meaning parent will whip said child off to a counsellor who will PERSUADE them that they are trans. Writing this now, it seems ridiculous, but honestly, I've had those comments directed at me.

When Leo and I did an interview for Sky News, I could not believe some of the comments I got about it on Twitter. (I can now see that Twitter seems to be almost nothing except a boiling pool of vitriol where everyone is maximally offended by everything, but also where everyone seems to think it's okay to speak to a person in a way that I can almost guarantee they would never do if they had to face that person in a room – why is that?) I had comments asking where Leo's father was (and for the record, we had been married about 20 years at that point). I had comments saying I was just an attention seeker. In fairness, thank God that most of the comments about Leo were just that he was "confused", "misled" and "misguided", rather than insulting him in the same hurtful way it was okay to insult me. Perhaps abusing a 16-year-old was just a step too far for some.

I've got off the point again and gone down a Twitter hole without even being on the app. My point was that most criticism seemed to suggest that Leo was just a tomboy "gone wrong". He wasn't.

Leo

Feeling wrong in my body wasn't really a thing for me when I was little. I didn't really think of it because as a young child, your main concerns are playing and having fun. You don't usually "develop a relationship with your body" or tend to think about it a great deal until you approach your teenage years. You don't yet understand how elements about yourself – e.g., your race, background, where you live or your appearance – intersect with and hold meaning in society, unless there are scenarios in which you're made to consider those things for some reason. You're yet to be socially conditioned to view your body as directly dictating and relating to your gender, sense of personhood and how you will be viewed by the world around you. All I knew when I was a child – more specifically, before I reached the age of ten – was that I just felt like a boy, and I didn't realize how that could be "wrong" or that I wasn't one.

As a young child, I dressed in a relatively masculine way (for a little girl), and was often assumed to be male by most people I interacted with. In public with my parents, strangers often spoke to me as if I was a little boy. It was so frequent, and every time a shop employee or stranger called me "mate" or said something to my parents about their "son", I lit up. It was a family inside joke for most of my childhood, as my parents were never offended and they could tell I liked it (for reasons none of us really understood or questioned at the time). So, when it happened, we all laughed along. In these moments I felt completely comfortable and entirely myself. I felt seen and experienced the thrill of knowing that no one "knew I was a girl". It wasn't until I began puberty that problems began to arise and the discomfort I felt about my female biology became overwhelming.

In primary school, my friends were mostly boys, and I hung around with who I wanted to and where I had the most fun, as kids do. I felt more like myself when I was with the other boys and always had a sense that amongst them was where I fit in. In clothes shops I was always attracted to the boys' section and anything masculine. Quite stereotypically, I didn't like pink. Even entering the girls' section, "just to look", as my mum sometimes encouraged me to do, felt wrong because if I did that, I was attaching myself to being a girl, admitting that the label fit me and facing the fact that that was how everyone saw me. And for reasons I couldn't understand or verbalize at the time, I wasn't able to allow it, for the same reason I never felt wholly comfortable with being referred to as a "tomboy" either. In school playgrounds my friends and I would play pretend families or make up sitcom-like scenarios in which I always played a man, usually called something like Jay for some reason (no offence to the Jays of the world, it just doesn't suit me). If we were pretending to be a family, I would be the husband and dad, and no one really questioned that a "girl" playing that role was factually incorrect because kids don't care, and we were all having fun regardless. Sometimes we'd play kiss chase, and I'd always be on the boys' team chasing the girls, or, when it was our time to run, I'd do so at a suspiciously slow pace. Being with the other boys was where I fit in, so though I had friends who were girls, I naturally drifted toward masculine things and people at nursery and primary school. It didn't occur to me at that time that I was the odd one out.

The key word that sums up how I felt when I started puberty is "alienated". I didn't have the language then to describe it in such a way, but I knew I felt like I was a boy and yet didn't have the body of one. As a pre-transition trans person, when all you ever see in the mirror and are told about yourself is the complete opposite to what you know you are, it's a shattering and isolating experience. And of course, that is where the motivation to transition derives from: to match your physical experience of yourself to the mental one.

It's important to note there are plenty of trans (including non-binary) people who don't feel the need or desire to medically transition – for them, being socially recognized as your chosen identity is affirming enough – but this has never been the case for me.

To try and explain gender dysphoria to someone who doesn't experience it – in other words, to someone who is cisgender – is tricky. The way I tend to articulate it is that when you're trans, the label of your sex assigned at birth never feels as if it truly fits you; and when you begin puberty and your body starts developing in what feels like the wrong way, it's definite that something is wrong. Some people like to use the metaphor that your body is "betraying you", which I can understand. The phrase describes the often-intense discomfort caused by the mismatch of how a person identifies and feels within themselves, compared to their sex assigned at birth and their physical self. It's a separation between mind and body, so the ways in which you experience your life and yourself can often feel inauthentic because your body, and therefore part of you, feels incomplete. If you feel like a man, but all you see when you look in the mirror are boobs, curves and female genitalia, it can be extremely distressing, and vice versa. You feel like your body is the wrong way around. The most accurate words to describe how experiencing gender dysphoria can feel are isolating, painful and alienating. It often seems that you can't escape it. You can bind, you can pack, you can tuck, but it's never what's truly there. You can't escape from your body. And you always know that. This makes dysphoria so troubling and overwhelming.

Despite the negative reactions and difficulties I faced at secondary school, I met people that made everything a hell of a lot easier. On my Year 6 "transition day" (haha), we visited the school we'd soon be joining in order to familiarize ourselves with the site and what our classes and peers would be like. During one textiles taster lesson, I spoke to a boy called Sam. Our first conversation was about the YouTubers "amazingphil" and "danisnotonfire", as we both subscribed to their channels. Once we began Year 7 together, we recognized each other and began talking again. Sam, I think, was the first person at my school I came out to because there was something about him that made me feel I was safe to do so, and I had a sense I didn't need to fear or worryingly anticipate his reaction. This is the same feeling I experience and look out for when meeting new people now, assessing if they are the kind of person I would ever tell. Ironically, he had heard about it before I told him, which proves my point about how fast it got around, but he was accepting and cool about it, nonetheless. He told me in one of our first conversations that he thought he might be bisexual but didn't know how to tell people or face it, and that became the first experience we bonded over. Sam and I hung out often, and he made me laugh more than anyone else I knew. For a little while I flitted between spending time with Sam and another friendship group, until I realized he was really the only person I felt I could be completely myself around. We spent most weekends and every second at school together. He very quickly became my best friend and the person I admired most. I would tell him every detail of what was going on in my life and update him about how things were going with my parents, how and when I got on waiting lists for the Tavistock and Portman gender clinic, and how every appointment went. We would comment on and insult the deliverers of every nasty remark we received and every difficult moment we'd face at school after he came out as gay and everyone knew I was trans. Almost a decade later, Sam is still my best friend, and our relationship has only grown stronger as we've grown up as queer men together, navigating things that few of the people around us could relate to or understand. It's accurate to say, and this is something that he knows full well, I don't know where I would be without him and our friendship.

Another difficulty during this time was when I started my menstrual cycle – it was a big thing. "Big" in the sense that I knew it was a part of womanhood and having periods meant I was going to become a woman. That realization evoked fear and immense anxiety for me. All I could think and worry about was, *How will I cope the more feminine I become?* Before puberty there were parts of my body that I didn't like. I hated. I didn't want them to be there. But I could still hide them under baggy clothes and hoodies, and people sometimes mistook me as a boy (due to being early on in puberty and not yet having a more feminine figure). Knowing that, in a few years, people would see me as a woman because I was shaped as one, because I had a feminine body, was such a distressing feeling. Even though puberty takes years, it continuously felt like I was already running out of time to stop it. *How am I going to live like this? I won't be able to do anything about it.* I felt that I was going to have to live as a woman my whole life, and at times I felt I'd rather not be here if that was to be the case.

To a degree, starting my periods meant I had to be more in touch with my body, and that was something that dysphoria didn't make easy. I always subconsciously managed to keep it separate in a way. I almost made it feel in my head that it wasn't part of me, because to have to face that fact every day or every time I got changed or showered would've been too exhausting and painful. That was something I spoke about a lot with my clinicians at Tavistock – how I didn't feel like certain parts of my body were mine and how I could never face the fact that they were. Luckily, my mum could see the effect it was having on me and how my mental health was deteriorating, so we agreed we should visit the GP and try to get me on the pill. Even though I knew this was something women did, it would stop my periods, and that was all that mattered to me. I make this point because, at this time in my life, *anything* feminine or traditionally associated with women would make me want to run a mile from it, but here I had to overlook that instinct of mine for my own benefit. My mum had gone on the pill when she was younger too, and this made her feel slightly better and more comfortable with the idea. Starting the pill didn't feel like a transition-related step as such – it was just something we could do to make sure

I wasn't so depressed and low, but nevertheless it made a great difference. At the time I wrote a diary entry about it. I used to write things down a lot, not for the purpose of showing anyone, but because it was a way to get some of the stuff out of my head that I didn't want to unload onto my parents. I knew they weren't ready to hear such depth and honesty about how I felt because it would upset and possibly confuse them, and all I wanted them to focus on was coming to terms with my trans-ness. I knew I'd be able to look back one day at the things I'd written and see how far I'd come and how different my position would be. Saying this, it's still hard for me to read my journal entries from times like that, despite it being so many years later, because as I look at the words, I remember just how alienated and scared I was:

Now this has happened, I feel less like a boy than I did before. I don't know how I'll be able to cope with the changes my body is going through.

Chapter 3

TELLING PEOPLE – COMING OUT AGAIN (AND AGAIN)

Gemma

Coming out wasn't just hard for Leo – it was hard for me, too. Not just because I was trying to deal with all my feelings about Leo being trans, understand what it would mean for him going forward and come to terms with everything I felt – grief, worry and like I'd "failed" in some way – but because I also had to come out to everyone on behalf of Leo, too.

I don't know why I don't remember this so well, but I can't recall the exact moment when I told my mum and dad – maybe because there wasn't an exact moment. My parents live in Spain, and although we are close and talk regularly, there's always a distance when important things are going on, which is difficult to cross. I don't think I spoke to them after the infamous coming-out night, for example, so I wouldn't have told them then. However, I would have broken the news sometime after that, certainly by the time we went to see the GP. Maybe my brain has just blocked that out, or maybe the menopause has just screwed my memory (and the rest of me at the same time!). When I very recently spoke to my mum about this, she doesn't remember a clear moment either. She said it had gradually become more obvious that there was "something" going on with Leo. But I guess because she'd seen some of our struggles over the years and seen Leo as a tomboy early on, there wasn't a big bombshell moment for her or my dad, which makes me feel a little bit better about my memory being dodgy.

However, I remember very clearly telling my brother and his wife. They live fairly close to us. They don't have kids themselves and are keen runners. I'd always felt a bit sad that they weren't close to our kids – because my parents were abroad, I felt like Leo and Luca missed out on a lot of the joy of an extended family, which I'd had when I was little. I spent a lot of time with my grandparents, especially in the holidays, and I think it's good for kids to have other adults they are close to. Anyway, I suspect it was a Sunday because I'd asked my brother if I could come and see them to talk about something, and they were out at a race. So, I drove along to it and met them both at the finish. It was a very odd discussion. Things were still raw for me, and I got quite upset. I remember sitting in this field on a blustery spring day, on plastic chairs near the refreshments tent with Piers and Niki fresh from their run, drinking a cup of tea and telling them all this momentous stuff. It felt weird being in such an ordinary setting and sharing life-changing news, with them all sweaty from their run.

I told them that E felt like she was a boy, that this was called being transgender, and we were going to support her moving forward and living as a boy. They seemed to take it much in their stride, with Piers even saying, "Well, it's not really a surprise, is it?" Maybe they had seen more than I had seen, I don't know, or perhaps it's just because they weren't that close to the kids, so it was easier for them to be more detached and objective. Of course, they did ask the same questions that lots of other people also went on to ask: "How can she be sure?", "What if she changes her mind?", "What does it actually mean … what will happen next?" I didn't have good answers for all those questions at that time. I did say that the statistics and research we'd done seemed to indicate that kids who thought they were trans, and continued to think that after puberty, were most likely trans and would be unlikely to change their minds.

Later on, Leo explained it to me in a great way, which I used a lot with other people. "Did you decide to be right-handed? Or did you decide to be straight? Or do you just know you 'are'? Well, that's what being trans is." Leo knew he was a boy. He knew in his body and in his heart. He wasn't deciding anything. Somehow, putting it in those terms made it easier for me, and for others, to understand how he felt. Anyway, they seemed to understand the choice that E had made and were happy to support it, which was the main thing. They didn't criticize; instead, they believed what I was saying, and they didn't change their opinion of E, or me, because of it. The reaction was positive – which I know isn't the case for many trans kids. I've heard of grandparents who refused to call a trans child by their new name or recognize the fact that they felt they were a different gender. I've even, heartbreakingly, heard the same about some parents. So, I felt sort of lucky that my family didn't judge or reject E or us. I drove away feeling relieved, but also exhausted and sad that this was cementing a reality that I still didn't feel ready for.

Someone else I clearly remember telling was my best friend, Teresa. I met up with her in London, and we went to the Pizza Express opposite Liverpool Street Station in the late afternoon. It was weird trying to be normal at first, even though she already knew there was something I wanted to talk to her about. She is a great listener and a great friend, and already had some experience of transgender issues. In fact, it was Teresa who originally told me about Mermaids, a charity that supports trans, non-binary and gender-diverse kids of all ages and their families – someone she knew had worked with the organization. So, with Teresa I could really open up and tell her everything I was feeling in a way I hadn't quite felt able to with my family. She is very open minded and accepting of people and difference, and she really helped me to pin down my feelings and worries with her calm and insightful questions. With other people I always felt a little bit like I was defending E's position and feelings and trying to explain on her behalf how she felt. I think that's because, in almost every case, I was the one with a bit more knowledge and understanding of things, whereas the people I was talking to were in the same position I had been when E first came out to us: they didn't really know what it meant and often had the same questions I'd had at first too.

But with Teresa, I told her that E had come out as transgender and that we'd been to the GP and were going to start counselling, but also that we were going to support her decision to live as a boy. I remember the poor waiter trying to take our order and bring out the food while ignoring the fact that I was basically crying my eyes out. I remember staring out of the window at all the people rushing by as he came over and letting Teresa do the ordering. It was the first time I'd really talked to someone else about everything: my worries about E choosing a life that would bring heartache, bullying, difficulty and prejudice, and how could I possibly choose or want that for my child; the worry about multiple surgeries and the risks associated with that; my ignorance of what being transgender meant, the fear of it all, of being different. *How would people, my family, adjust to E being a boy? How on earth could I go about telling people?*

Teresa got me to explain my worries one by one and helped me see that although it wouldn't be easy, there were positives. The positives were that E was in a loving, supportive family; any surgery was years away and could be taken step by step; and E would become happier, as she started to live the life she wanted. Teresa reminded me that it was okay to be transgender – people dealt with it every day – and that by starting earlier, it would make the process much easier than it was for people who came out late in life, sometimes with marriages and children behind them. And as I mentioned before, she said there were organizations that could help, and that most importantly, she and others would be there for E, for me and for our family. I don't think I had cried so much for years. It was partly relief about being able to say everything, honestly, out loud. It was partly relief that maybe I had been catastrophizing. And it was also a realization that we just had to take one step at a time – that surgery was a long way away, and that not all trans people even had surgery! I think for the first time I had a sense of hope for the future, that it needn't be as "bad" as I had envisioned it to be, that there could be upsides. I realized that we all had the strength to get through it. I left that Pizza Express with a red, puffy face, a massive headache and a huge hug from Teresa.

Weirdly, the next big place to "come out" again for me was at work. I had taken a "proper" job again after a period of running my own marketing agency. I made this decision for two reasons: firstly, the agency had faltered as I struggled to simultaneously run it and come to terms with what was happening with our family life; and secondly, I realized that I needed the headspace to adapt and be more available for E and our family. With my new job, I was back in an office again, working in the City in London. Luckily, even though this was before the Covid-19 pandemic, I didn't have to go in every day, but I did go in a couple of days a week. My boss, Heather, lived in Scotland, so I got to see her in person a couple of times a month. She was great – a really warm, empathetic and authentic person – and I really liked working with her. The company was great too, and I met some people there who I really connected with and I'm still in touch with today.

Nevertheless, I did find it hard in the office when talking about my eldest child. I found that I would automatically start sentences with, "Oh, when my oldest was a baby/at school/etc.", because I was trying to avoid pronouns. It still felt a bit weird thinking of my son when, in the memories I was sharing, he was my daughter, so I just tried to avoid it.

But eventually, I started to feel safer, and Leo's transition had started to progress. I knew we were only going one way with what was happening and felt that the best thing to do would be to start being open about it. So, in a meeting with Heather, I decided to take the plunge and tell her. I had to occasionally take Leo for appointments at Tavistock, the doctor's or other places, and of course, when you start having to do that regularly, it feels dishonest not to be able to say why. People are usually concerned enough to ask why you're taking your child to the doctor's, or at least they tend to ask, "I hope it's nothing serious?"

Heather was great though – super supportive, and although she didn't pretend to know much about what was going on beyond the basics that most people at the time knew, she asked important and open questions and made me realize that it would be okay to share more with people. Because I work in the tech sector, a lot of my connections and colleagues are on LinkedIn, and I'd been on it for years too. So, in much the same way as I'd announced Leo to the world on Facebook to my family and friends, I chose LinkedIn as the platform to announce this to my network, too. LinkedIn isn't meant to be a platform for sharing personal news so much, and back then it was even more unusual than it is now. But I wrote a blog about Leo coming out and how badly I'd handled it, but how important it was, and I posted it there for the world to see. Not for the first or last time, I had a great response. (When I posted on LinkedIn that we were writing this book, and it was being published, I had the most amazing and life-affirming responses.) People I knew well commented and sent me messages, and colleagues even plucked up the courage in the lift to the office, or in the kitchen, to let me know that they saw my post, and "by the way – well done". It was a huge weight off my mind, and I started to feel able to share more about Leo and our journey with people in a work environment. What was really lovely, too, was the number of trans people, or people with trans kids or relatives, who messaged me. They nearly always did so privately, but they empathized, were grateful to me for speaking out and always had positive messages to share. I really cherished each one, and I guess it's part of the reason why I felt convinced to share our story with a wider audience and write this book. Leo and I really just hope that some people will pick up our story and it will help them in some way – give them a new insight, understanding or just a bit of recognition for what they, their family, friends or colleagues might have gone through.

Once I'd told the closest people to us, and everyone at work, I decided, with Leo and Bill's approval, to then post it on Facebook so that everyone knew, and I didn't have to keep having the same conversation over and over. This is my post:

3 SEPTEMBER 2017

Hello! It's me. Some of you may remember (and some may just not have noticed) that I gave up Facebook in January as my New Year's Resolution. I have a confession to make … I have been using FB since then, but only as part of a private group. Now seems like a good time to make the reasons for joining that private group public, and to share something with you all, as the new school year will mean some big changes for our family.

This September, E will be going back to school as Leo. About a year ago, Leo told us he was transgender. For those of you who don't really know what that means (and I didn't), it means that Leo has always felt like a boy trapped in the body of a girl. A lot of things made sense – E was never a very girly girl. We always used to argue because she always made me buy boys' clothes and all sorts of other things.

Safe to say, the last year has been a tumultuous one for us all, as we've struggled to come to terms with what in the beginning felt to us like we were losing our daughter and, in turn, trying to understand what must be going through the mind of our son as he has struggled to cope with these feelings and changes himself. We've had many difficult, often tearful conversations with each other. Some months ago, we joined the FB group for an organization called Mermaids, and they've been brilliant. We've met other families with trans kids, in person and online, and it's become clear that not only are we not alone, but that transgender children are everywhere – we've found two other families in Bedford. To some people I know, this might just seem like a trend – certainly I'd never heard the term "transgender" growing up. But to me, it feels like this is something that people are finally being able to say and choose, much in the same way as people just a few decades ago were first able to come out and openly say they were gay. I'd highly recommend Mermaids as a place to go if you'd like to find out more.

We've got to a place now, led by Leo, who has shown maturity, understanding and patience with us way beyond his years, where we've agreed that the school can use Leo as his given name, as many of his friends have been doing for months.

The future will hold a whole series of other changes, as we'll be attending the Tavistock Centre in London next year, the only place that assesses children for gender transition. If that all goes according to plan, Leo will then be offered hormone blockers, a reversible treatment that puts puberty on hold. Until he is 16, he will be assessed physically and mentally to ensure he is really committed and 100 per cent sure of his feelings, and then he will be given testosterone, which will start the hormonal process of making him more outwardly a man.

Up to this point and beyond, I could not be prouder of our son – the strength he has shown in sharing with us his feelings, dealing with our struggles to accept them, and bravery in facing the future. I wanted to share this news with everyone here. We've had some conversations with some of you individually, and I thank those of you for your support. Sometimes though, a point comes where you just want to put the news "out there" – so here it is. Thanks for listening.

* * *

Leo

After coming out to my parents and friends, my parents and I waited until we felt ready, and then we decided it was time to tell our extended family. This was largely something they took on – not because I didn't want to, but because we all felt it would make more sense for my parents to tell the relatives, as they would have the opportunity to ask my parents things that they may not have wanted to ask in front of me, so the conversations could go into greater depth. I was happy with this because I trusted them to speak well on my behalf and accurately portray how I felt. My mum told my older half-brothers (my dad's other sons), who were both incredibly supportive, though they said it was a surprise. I recently found the text messages from the conversation with my eldest brother Mike, when I asked him if Mum had spoken to him about it yet. Below is a snippet:

Mike: *I think it'll take me a bit of time to get used to, but I will over time. I'm happy for you that you know what you want, and I'm pleased you're going through with it. If it's what makes you happy, then I'm happy too.*

Me: *Thank you, Mikey. Love you.*

Mike: *Love you too, Leo.*

As far as I remember, we told our family members in dribs and drabs, whenever we saw them or decided it was an appropriate time to do so. We were very pleased and lucky to not receive any overly negative reactions from those we came out to. This, of course, isn't the case as often as it should be for trans people – plenty lose relationships with members of their families through their decision to transition, or as a result of being open about their identities. Often, when someone not as close to us in my extended family was informed, they didn't find it surprising. This was the case with my mum's brother and his wife, who both replied to my mum with words to the effect of, "Well ... is it really a big shock? Look what he was like when he was younger," and so on. My dad's mum, who was in her seventies at the time, a traditional Italian woman who migrated to England in the 1950s, had no issue or qualms with the news nor the changing of my name, and in fact picked up the change in pronouns and how she addressed me very quickly. Though she had to get her head round it initially, this has remained the case, as she is fully aware of my medical transition and has always been so accepting about it, which I find slightly astounding at times. Her memory never fails her (except for the instances in which she forgets I'm pescetarian and makes me ham sandwiches when I go to visit her, but we work around it).

My mum's parents initially found the news trickier to comes to terms with, and for a short while, they had a tougher time adjusting to my new pronouns. I think the difficulty for them came from the fact that they are closer to us as a family than my dad's mum. But as with everyone, whenever they'd make a mistake or misgender me, they would realize and apologize quickly, so I was never offended. It occasionally catches me off guard even now to see and hear my grandparents refer to me as their grandson, considering their ages and what life was like for trans people during the period in which they were born. I feel incredibly privileged to have the supportive and loving family I was born into. An important thing to note is that when people are adjusting to someone's new name or pronouns, they're bound to make mistakes early on. They're changing behaviours that, in some cases, are decades old, so it's to be expected. As long as there's respect, and they correct themselves when they realize that they've misgendered you, then they're doing all they can.

The person who was really the pioneer of accepting me in our family was my little brother, Luca. He was very young when I came out, perhaps seven or eight when we first explained to him what was going on, although we, of course, didn't go into great detail. There was no point yet to get into specifics with him or discuss what might happen to me physically in the future because he didn't need to know that to accept it. The thing is, as is often remarked on but it is certainly true, kids don't care. Children are not intrinsically biased or hateful toward anyone; these are behaviours and reactions they learn. As he got older, he knew me as his brother and was the first person in the house to call me Leo. His almost blind, unquestioning acceptance, which probably stemmed from the fact he was a child and wasn't yet aware of the complicated conventions and construct of gender, was crucial for me in feeling like there was someone around me who I didn't have to struggle against. He now knows about everything we discuss in this book and understands that it was hard time I went through with our parents. He has said to me before that it doesn't feel odd knowing that I was once "his sister" because now I've been his brother for longer, and he feels that I've always been Leo to him. We have always been close and now he's older, 17 by the time this is published, I couldn't be more grateful for his enduring and everlasting support. Love you, Lulu.

Being completely out to my friends and family felt as if a weight had been lifted off my shoulders. I no longer carried the burden of being known by my old name, and instead felt free from having to hide part of myself around certain people and in certain situations. I was Leo to everyone, and that allowed me to blossom in confidence as I entered young adulthood. All that was left for me to focus on were the next steps in my transition.

Chapter 4

BETWEEN

Gemma

It's safe to say that those first few months after E came out were the hardest I've ever experienced, and I've experienced few other things I wouldn't wish on my worst enemy. I'm just sharing these awful and embarrassing examples of my lack of understanding and poor behaviour to try and demonstrate some of the turmoil of emotions we've been through. I also hope to show that, although sometimes I was about as far away as it's possible to get from being an understanding, supportive parent through this transition, by some miracle we got through it. And more than that – Leo and I have become much closer than I thought we could when I envisaged that bright, shiny future with a daughter. I realize this is mainly entirely due to him, his strength, sensitivity and all-round awesomeness, but without going through this awful pain, I genuinely don't think we'd have the relationship we have now or feel like we could both share all this stuff with other people.

In this next section, I call Leo "she" still because that's how I felt at the time. At that point, I hadn't accepted Leo as himself and still thought I had a daughter – albeit one who was changing. Even writing this still feels weird putting "she". But again, at that time, it was the pronoun I was still using (sorry, Leo).

I remember one of the times that E and I were talking in the car and I was trying to explain the grief I felt about her transition in a way that made sense. I told her that I felt like I was "losing my daughter". I was so sad; it was almost like the person I knew as E was dying and I was being left behind. I was so overwhelmed with my own pain and sadness that there was so much I didn't see from her point of view.

We seemed to have endless discussions about it all. I was trying to be as open as I could and listen to my child, but as I shared my pain with E, she was the parent at times. "Mum, you're doing really well. I know you are trying to come to terms with it. I know how hard it is." It's still hard to think about the selfishness of putting my feelings onto my 12-year-old child and the incredible generosity of her response. But I felt that I had to be totally open – and I do think it helped us get to a better place eventually, even though it was so hard to do. In some ways I felt so overwhelmed. Sometimes I know I wanted E to understand the pain I felt, and sometimes I even wanted to inflict it on her, as if she didn't have enough to cope with.

Puberty was the thing that really made us realize we had to act, accept what our child was telling us and let the future take its course. Weirdly, one thing I remember thinking that made me (even more) worried about "letting" E transition was the fact that I thought this was a never-going-back thing. That I was "letting" E make changes that would affect her for the rest of her life – that she would never, ever be able to step back from what she was deciding to do now. And I panicked. I thought she was too young for such a weighty "decision". I felt like I couldn't leave that burden with her. All wrong. Of course, all those things are wrong!

I realize that a lot of people I talk to, especially those that have never met a trans person or don't really understand the issues, still think that being trans is a decision. I realize that a lot of the absolute crap I see on Twitter largely stems from this. People think kids are being "radicalized" into thinking that they are trans. People have blamed the Tavistock Centre for "pandering" to the whims of overly politically correct parents who are "allowing" (in some cases, I've even heard it called "encouraging") their kids to be trans. There's all this shit about there only being two genders, that you're male or female and that's it. I've been accused of harming my child, of Munchausen's by proxy for letting my child "mutilate" himself.

So let me just address some of that stuff head on.

I get it.

I get why people are worried that kids can't make these decisions.

I get why they're worried that parents are letting them change their lives in difficult and potentially dangerous ways.

I get it because THAT IS HOW I FELT TOO.

I was scared. I didn't want E to transition. I was worried sick! I was worried she'd be unhappy, that she would be the victim of discrimination for her whole life. That she would never find love. That she would have to undergo painful and delicate surgery.

It took a very long time to accept E's transition, to be ready to start having those conversations. And why and how I got there was because of E herself. Her absolute bravery of having the realization that she was different – looking it up on the internet, discovering what "transgender" meant and working out that it was what she was. Then, her decision to try and share this with us, and her heart-breaking realization that we didn't get it, and although we tried, were not supporting her in the way she wanted or needed. I'm still unable to comprehend the amount of strength that must have taken.

I finally realized, in E's case, there was no "letting" her be anything – she already WAS herself. She wasn't asking my permission to change. She wasn't deciding anything. She WAS a boy. It took me *soooo* long to see and understand that. In one of our many conversations when I was upset and sad, I remember trying to explain how I felt, and E said to me, "Mum, if this wasn't something I had to do, do you think I'd be putting us all through this?"

It was one of the moments that really helped me understand how she felt. That it wasn't a change she was making – she was just being herself. It's just that she wasn't who we all originally thought she was.

Once we finally started to accept that E was turning into Leo, things got a little bit easier. After seeing the GP, then going to the Child and Adolescent Mental Health Services (CAMHS), then Tavistock, and with things changing at school, Leo started to emerge as himself. He took tentative steps at first perhaps, but made bolder changes with clothes, haircuts and behaviour.

To start off with, Leo presented as hyper-masculine. I thought he felt that, after all the heartbreak, questions and counselling, there was no room to be anything else. That to be anything other than the most masculine version of himself was to somehow be unconvincing or "not trans enough". But I'm jumping ahead.

After E came out, for a while it felt like every discussion we were having was about being transgender. It was like a huge boil had been lanced for E, and all of a sudden, I guess for her, she was finally able to make sense of how she felt, and also was naturally curious about every aspect of being transgender. One thing that really helped her was watching some early pioneers on YouTube who posted every aspect of their own journeys – warts and all. It really helped E to see people like her talking openly about their feelings, how hard they were finding everything, and sharing the reactions they had had in their own lives to coming out, being transgender and being accepted (and sometimes, not being accepted) by their friends, families and schoolmates. Those brave individuals really were trailblazers, and although they could see some of their impact through the comments on their posts, I wonder if they even really understood how much they were helping others by sharing their own struggles.

We were trying to be supportive, but we were also finding it so difficult to talk about all the time. I know it took Bill longer to come to terms with, and for him it was even more difficult. I remember him telling me that he had always wanted a girl (he had two older boys before Leo and Luca), and he was heartbroken to "lose" E. I felt the same, and there was a real sense of grief about "losing" a daughter. It was only when we went to family counselling at CAMHS, as recommended by our GP, that one of the counsellors explained these feelings of grief in a way that started to make sense.

The counsellor explained that it was kind of like a mourning for a future we had imagined but had lost. The constant conversations with E were draining. It was making me face up to the facts full on, and I felt like I had nowhere to go. I couldn't leave it aside or pretend it wasn't happening, and it was very hard. I remember we would often talk in the car because it was a space where we were together and had the time to do so. One day I remember asking E if we could talk about something else for a change. Again, I didn't realize then how much she needed to talk about everything and how hard it must have been for her. There were a good few months of this "in-between" stage, when although we loved and supported E, it felt like the transition hadn't properly "started" or been allowed to start, and we were all feeling our way along what was, at times, a very bumpy path.

One bump on that path was Leo's new name. Choosing a new name surely has to be a highlight of being transgender. After all, haven't we all at some time wanted to be called something else? In my late teens, I went through a phase of wishing I'd been given a different name – something "cooler". Of course, as a child of the '70s and '80s, what was cool then potentially would very much not be the same now! So, with apologies to anyone called by any of these names – I'm sure you're much cooler than I am – I toyed with formally changing my name to Skye (which I still love), Scarlett or Sidney. Ironically, I didn't even think about the confusion that might be created by being a girl and then a young woman called Sidney. (I wonder if I would have been more or less successful in job interviews if people thought I was a man when they asked me to come in. Probably a topic for another day.)

Anyway, once we eventually got our heads around the fact that Leo felt like a boy, truly was a boy and was going to start living as a one, then of course he had to think of a new name. He tried to think of a few alternatives, but Robert was the only other name that was really in contention. Sorry to any Roberts, but I really can't imagine him as a Robert. (What even does a Robert look like? For some reason, in my head, a Robert has to have dark hair. I don't know why I think that!) But once he settled on Leo, it seemed to fit him well. There were certainly the connotations of strength and bravery that come with choosing the name of a lion, and he'd shown buckets of both. Plus, it felt like a name to be proud of. So, Leo it was.

Of course, I say that like it was all decided, simple and easy, and we all switched to calling him Leo immediately. It was absolutely nothing like that. First, it was almost impossible to stop calling him E – especially when shouting from the kitchen that dinner was ready, or asking Luca to "ask ... *ah, dammit* ... see what you both want for dinner ..." I became an expert in sentences that avoided the need for both a name and pronouns. I would go up to Leo instead of shouting (like a good parent should anyway), and say, "What do you want to do/have for dinner/etc.?" I would try to avoid naming my child in public. I would say "my son ...", rather than his name, to work colleagues. All sorts of tricks. Bill settled on "Muppet". You might think that sounds a bit harsh, but for most of our married life, we've called each other "Spoon". I don't know where that came from either, but Muppet at least meant Bill could address Leo directly without the need for the stupid evasive sentences that I was using. Bill still occasionally calls Leo "Muppet"; Leo and I call each other "Bro" or "Broski" to this day. We do it literally all the time – in texts, in shops, at work. I do admit that I quite like it when someone looks surprised that I'm calling this young man "Bro". And for us, it's a term of endearment, although I also have no idea where it came from.

Luca was the first person in our family to call Leo by his name. Perhaps this massive change for all of us came more naturally to him, as he was only around eight or nine at the time, but he never seemed to struggle with things in the way that we did. If someone asked him, he would say, "I used to have a sister, but now I have a brother." Like it was no big deal to him. He didn't feel the need to overexplain and otherwise just didn't even mention it. Sam, Leo's best friend at school, started calling him "Lur", which was kind of a cross between the name E and Leo. I tried calling him "Lur" for a bit too, but it just felt really awkward. Gradually, his friends at school switched to calling him Leo, which meant that the conversation with school came up fast.

I remember clearly deciding to tell Leo that we were ready to make the change official. It was in the summer holiday, between Years 7 and 8, around 18 months after he first told us about being trans, and that awful conversation in his bedroom. We'd all travelled a long way since then, and it was a pretty momentous decision. Leo and I had been waiting for a time when his dad felt able to deal with it. So, when Bill got home, I called Leo into my office and told him, "Next year you can go back to school as Leo." I showed him the name change certificates I'd created. (These are dead simple. Mermaids helped us, but basically you just need to say that from now on, you want to be known as this name. You don't need to do it "officially" online or anything – that's certainly worth knowing. You basically just have to decide to do it.) He was SO happy. He started to cry. I started to cry (obviously). Even Bill shed a few tears. It was a real moment of validation for Leo, and one that had taken a long time to get to. It was key milestone in his transition for all of us.

So, we officially changed Leo's name everywhere – at the doctor's, who were happy to make the change and knew of the situation anyway. At the dentist, who was brilliant and super supportive. With bank accounts, his child trust fund, and of course, we applied for a new passport. Leo's formal transition was underway and now felt "official".

* * *

Leo

The reason the title of this book is *Between* is because that word is painfully suited to much of what we as a family, and I as an individual, went through after I came out. Much of the time following my coming out, before I socially transitioned, was spent in between names, waiting lists, identities and progress. For so long, my parents couldn't grasp the situation, accept me as their son or understand quite what I wanted and needed my future to look like. Initially, it was the concept of being transgender that they wrestled with. As many people don't realize, the choice for us isn't to *be* trans, it's to *transition*. (And even that, in a physical sense, isn't a path all trans people wish to take.) For all of us, though, there's not much about it that feels like a choice. This chapter reflects on how my identity intersected with the things going on in my life – before I socially transitioned and began living fully as myself.

At first, teachers still had to call me my old name. They wouldn't change the registers or call me anything different without my parents' approval, which was understandable, and I wouldn't have asked for that without them being involved. However, this meant that, for a while, I was going by multiple names within different groups of people during Years 7 and 8. My close friends called me Leo. For most of Year 7, people at school who didn't know I was trans called me E. Dad then started calling me "Muppet" and avoiding pronouns, and toward the end of the school year, teachers had me as "L" on the register and addressed me as such. This was a compromise agreed on by my parents and me. It meant I didn't have to see or have a relationship to my old name directly, but there wasn't a complete separation from my deadname and previous pronouns. For a while, Mum called me L because it was a non-gendered term, and I didn't feel as if she was calling me my old name, though she did try to avoid pronouns where possible, but we both knew it didn't sound right. Thinking back, the way my dad referred to me is actually quite funny – literally everything would be, "That's Muppet's," or, "Where's Muppet?" – and that name has stuck (although in jest – he does address me as Leo and has done for years). Muppet was just my name for a good chunk of that year for my dad, and of course I preferred it to the alternative. After that, there was a time when my mum and Luca were calling me Leo, whilst Dad was still using Muppet. It's fair to say the confusion and variance between how I was viewed and spoken to over that time sums up just how awkward and painful socially transitioning can be.

It was in the summer of Year 7, before I joined Year 8, that my parents decided that I could go back to school as Leo. In the weeks before I was told this could finally be the case, I knew that Mum had come a long way with it all. She was adapting to my new name and pronouns, and every day she made fewer mistakes – it started to sound more natural to us all. On the other hand, because of his inward and stoic nature, I had no idea how my dad was feeling about everything. He was always reluctant to talk about his feelings about anything, but being clueless about what he felt at any given time was especially hard then. He was calling me Muppet and quite successfully avoiding pronouns, but there was never, in the years after me coming out, a *single* conversation between him and I about where he was at or when he might be ready for me to change my name. I felt as if I was in limbo. I never wanted to put pressure on my parents, despite how desperately I needed and wanted everything to change, because I wanted things to change when *they* were ready, not because I'd pushed them into it too early for them to cope with.

Year 7 was my first year at my secondary school, and it was a tough year because of the variance in levels of acceptance I felt from those around me. It had been over a year since I came out to my parents, and I often felt hopeless that my transition was never going to go the way I desperately wanted it to go. I recently found a diary entry dated 27 June 2016, in which I wrote:

Dear future Leo,
There will be a day when Dad understands,
There will be a day when he calls you his son,
There will be a day when you're complete.

After the summer of Year 7, before I went into Year 8, Mum and Dad told me I could go back to school as Leo. At that point my name wasn't legally changed (this happened later – in April 2017, in the middle of Year 8), but they were prepared to let me be recognized by my chosen name and pronouns by my peers and the school administration. It seemed to my parents that if we were going to make the change, doing so before the start of the academic year was the most appropriate time. Plus, I'm sure they knew that waiting another year to do this would've been unbearable for me. Mum has told me, during the process of writing this book, that she and Dad had many difficult conversations about it. Without pressuring him, and though she might not have been wholly ready herself for such a big change to occur, she helped him realize that how I felt wasn't going to go away. Mum recalls telling me how she told Dad, "You know this is the right thing to do." She told me, "We both loved you. We both knew how difficult it was for you." And that it was especially a massive thing for Dad to be able to accept me as Leo. Massive for him, and massive for me.

One day during the summer holidays, we were at home, and I was in the living room. Dad got home from work, and Mum called me into the room she was in, so I went, not thinking twice about why. As I entered, she was standing in front of me. She was pulling a kind of face that looked mischievous and she was smiling. I got the feeling that whatever she was going to tell me was going to be exciting. She explained that she'd spoken to Dad about it, and they were ready for me to go back to school as Leo. I asked, "Are you sure Dad's okay with it?" She nodded, and I burst into tears. It was the first time since I'd come out, almost two years before, that I had received any validation and a sense of understanding from my dad. It meant more to me than I can describe. Mum had obviously told him that she was about to have the conversation with me because when I practically ran into the kitchen to hug him, with tears streaming out of my eyes, he just squeezed me back and said, "It's okay, Muppet."

The next step was to find out how to go about changing my name. It wasn't a process I knew much about, especially as most of the trans guys whose YouTube videos I watched online were American, so their process was entirely different. I didn't know many people first-hand who'd done it. Not long after that, we found out from Mermaids how to get my name changed. It luckily wasn't as complicated as we worried it would be. You don't have to do it legally as such, but there is set wording that helps. We printed that off on certificate-type paper and sent it to everyone – the doctors and the dentists and the people in charge of my bank account, and everyone else that needed to be informed. The hard part was just explaining my situation to so many people and institutions to get them to alter their records for me. We also had to apply for a new passport with my new name and the "M" sex marker. I was lucky in that my mum navigated all this stuff for me – she is very much the "doer" in the family.

I was worried that we would run into problems accessing a new passport. The last time we'd gone on holiday, to visit my grandparents who live in Spain, we had multiple awkward moments where the officer checking my passport pulled a face and did a double take at my passport because they were reading, "E Telford, F", but looking at a 13-year-old boy. It was always excruciatingly embarrassing somehow to explain, "Oh, yep, that's me, haha. Definitely a girl, I just look like I boy! I get it all the time, haha!" There was no point getting into the actual details because there was never time, and what was the point? This wasn't going to happen anymore eventually, and I'd rather not have to come out to the airport check-in staff or a passport officer in front of a queue of hundreds of people.

When my name was changed, everything was so much easier – not just in the legal sense, but I felt lighter. The first few times going to the dentist was awkward because they'd known me as E for so long, but it got easier. After my name was changed, for a long time, I worried about what those people thought about it. I wondered if they even *did* think about it. I was sure they did – trans people weren't as well understood or present anywhere at the time, or so it seemed, so I was certain people like the doctor and dentist had their own thoughts on the matter. I used to fret about whether they thought I was "too young" to be making such a "big decision", or that my parents were foolish for letting a "confused child get their way". All these things were based on ignorant comments all too commonly directed at trans kids and their parents, and I suppose I had internalized them. Plus, I was younger, so I was more prone to caring what people think. But the truth was, everyone just got used to it. And now, I care very little about what people think of me or my parents' decisions because I know they are probably just not that educated on the matter and have no real understanding of the kind of things we and families like us go through.

As I'm sure you have gathered, there was (what felt to me like) a long time of being *between* everything in my life – between names; between transitioning, acceptance and comfort; and ultimately, between where my mental health had been in the beginning of the journey and happiness. For this period, it felt that the cloud of my coming out and trans identity hung over me. And not just me, but my family as well. It was inescapable. For my mum and me, it felt like we couldn't hang out, talk or enjoy each other's company properly, as long as it was there. And it always was. It felt to me that in every interaction between us, the elephant in the room stood in the corner. I knew it was always in the back of our heads, and for a while, if I brought it up, or spoke about something related to it, it caused upset and ruined whatever we were doing.

It was certainly the case for a lot of this period in my life and transition that I felt as if I was the parent to my parents. This sounds harsh to say, and of course I don't mean that I tackled all the responsibilities and stresses that a parent has, but for a 12 and 13-year-old, I had the mindset and burden of protecting and caring for and reassuring my parents, which no child should feel they have to do. My mum would agree that this dynamic played out mainly between her and I, as we were the ones who communicated the most, always open and honestly, about how we were feeling regarding everything. My dad isn't a man for communicating particularly well, hence his exclusion here.

I felt this way the most after a heated conversation that Mum and I had in the car together. These situations always took place in the car for some reason. (I've been told that the best time to have hard or difficult talks is while walking or driving with someone because the lack of eye contact takes the pressure off what you say, which I think sounds plausible.) Anyway, I don't remember how we got to talking about me and trans stuff, but Mum began to get upset and asked if we could talk about something else. I tried to make clear to her that that was hard for me because I knew she didn't want to hear it, but in my head, it was such a pressing issue, and I spent so much of my own time thinking about it. She didn't have anything to say, so for the rest of the journey, we sat in silence, unable to think of the right way to break the silence and lighten the mood or reassure each other without upsetting ourselves. When we got home, Luca and Dad were out. As soon as she put her stuff down, she walked hastily upstairs and into her room. I knew she had gone to let herself cry. I shortly followed her, and as I opened the door, she was perched on her bed, sobbing into her hands that covered her face. For a few minutes, neither of us said anything, and I hugged her. Although how she (and my dad) was feeling was hurting me so much, I couldn't let her be so upset, especially knowing I was the cause. This, in turn, inspired guilt in me whenever I thought about it. I hugged her and told her it would get easier. She cried more and shook her head. I knew that, at that moment, she couldn't see a time when she would ever be able to let go of E and all that she meant to her. She lifted her head and told me, "I feel like I'm grieving, like you've died. I feel like I'm losing my daughter."

I knew she was struggling, but I was too, and I know she knew this. However, she was so caught up with her own struggles that she couldn't yet comprehend my problems or make herself present to console me. Writing this book has made me realize how hard I find remembering moments like these, moments that weren't as infrequent as I'd hoped they would be. I am sure this is partly due to the fact I've managed to push most these memories out of my mind and block them out, so I don't often have to contemplate or feel them again.

Though I made good friends in Year 7, and at first was swept away with joining a new, big school, all I can really recall from that year is how low and hopeless I felt. By the end of the year, things were looking up – we were seeing CAMHS and I was on the waiting list for Tavistock – but my memory of this "between" period is dominated by my low spirits, and I genuinely struggle to recollect and think back to much of that year at school.

Something that helped me feel less alone during this time were the trans content creators I came across online. They are certainly more abundant now, due to the fact it's safer and more generally socially acceptable to be visible now than it was when I started transitioning. But back then, I was still able to find trans men online who spoke openly and honestly about their experiences and transitions, which was invaluable to me. Finding them allowed me to realize there were more trans people in the world than I thought, and that, in turn, helped me feel like maybe I wasn't as different as I felt. It gave me a sense of community and belonging, despite geographical boundaries. Some of people I followed on Instagram included the American bodybuilder Ajay Holbrook, who was a big inspiration for me, as since the start of my teenage years, I've been interested in fitness and working out. On YouTube, I watched videos by Alex Bertie and his "The Quest to Alex's Beard" series. Watching Ajay and Alex's content made me so excited and hopeful for what was to come in the future, after my medical transition – and looking back on this now can make my life as it is now feel so surreal.

Shortly after coming out and for years after, I felt a constant pressure to be hyper-masculine. The pressure was partly from my own insecurity of feeling that I wasn't as masculine as I wanted to present and feel, but also from the assumption that the more "straightforward" and manly I was as a trans person, the easier I would be for people to understand, and the more respected and less harassed I might be. Of course, admitting this now is sad and sort of embarrassing, but fitting and moulding yourself to please other people and their expectations is something I think we all do, especially my fellow trans and queer people, particularly earlier on in our lives. It can be out of fear, anxiety and necessity. The slightly funny thing is that I am still what most would categorize as a typically "masculine" man. I dress exclusively in men's clothes, have had short hair my whole teenage and adult life, and don't have features stereotypically associated with women or femininity. But the standard I set myself in Year 7 and Year 8 was ridiculous. I would hate hearing my voice naturally reach higher pitches when exclaiming or talking in conversation with others, so I would make an effort for my voice to be at a low pitch at all times. I would constantly be hyper-aware of how I walked, sat and talked, in order to present as the most macho person in the room. I feared that any sense of femininity would somehow discredit my transness and give people permission to no longer take me seriously. It took years for this pressure to wear off, but it did – eventually. What is ironic is the fact that I knew how harsh and silly I was being. I knew full well that no matter how I dressed or behaved, nothing made a difference.

As a reaction to the way I'd suppressed myself previously, between the ages of 15 to 16, I very briefly experimented with wearing makeup and different clothes. This came about as I started to accept my queerness in ways other than just the fact that I'm trans. I never went out in public with makeup on, but there was one time I posted a picture to Instagram of my face wearing some sort of eye makeup in what I thought was some sort of political statement (LOL – I was a child, okay?), and I felt confident and defiant in doing so. This lasted maybe a matter of weeks, as I decided that although it would be totally fine if this was how I wanted to present, I discovered it just wasn't my thing. I am better being a plain-looking guy, but I'm pleased I gave myself space to explore different expressions of my identity.

Chapter 5

NAVIGATING SCHOOL

Gemma

Leo was the first transgender kid at his school. We're not saying that because we've got some inflated sense of importance about it – we're saying it because everyone at the school told us that, and this meant they had to do a lot of learning about how to handle it.

Coming out at school was tough for E, and then Leo, and it was perhaps the between-est bit of being between E and Leo. It literally was making the transition transparent to everyone, and it was a jumbly, awkward period of changes that we all adapted to at different speeds. The school had no more idea about what to do with E than we did, really, but the staff were open to supporting her and us, although at times it was a little like the blind leading the blind.

E started secondary school in Year 7, and in that year, was still known at school as E. However, she had already come out to her friends, and her friendship group, including Sam, her best friend, were open and supportive, as I've discovered so many teenagers are. As a group, kids are much more accepting of transgender kids (there are always some exceptions, which we'll come to), and they're respectful of people's choice when it comes to their gender and pronouns. Because E hadn't officially become Leo at that point, there was also an in-between-ness about names. Still E at home, she became "Lur" to Sam, which was kind of in between

E and Leo, or just Leo. Physically, E started to change how she was presenting to the outside world much more, with shorter, more boyish hair, and more boyish clothes to match. There was a tight-knit group of friends who used to hang out together, and they were a great support for E/Leo.

Our first meeting was with E's head-of-year and form tutor. We trooped into the teaching block and sat with her on the scratchy, hard chairs seemingly beloved by institutions everywhere. She was a well-meaning person, but really had no idea of what to do or say. And of course, she'd had no training – all of this was new to her – so why should we have expected her to handle it any better than we had? We went in to see her and explained that, although it was difficult, we supported E's decision to change her name and pronouns, but we weren't quite ready for that to be official – yet. It was a bit of a weird, upsetting conversation, and emotions were still raw for us all at that point. We told her that we accepted that Leo was transgender, that we'd been to see the GP, that we were on the waiting list for Tavistock, that we'd started seeing CAMHS, and that this had been a painful, difficult period for us all.

We did manage to get some practical changes agreed, which helped in this weird in-between period. E would have access to a toilet and changing room that was individual and gender neutral. She was given a key for it, and it was more or less available just for her. That solved the changing room and toilet question in one easy step. Then, in terms of sports, E could just pick which sports she wanted to be a part of. Some sports were mixed anyway, and in others she could choose how she participated. Dance and cheerleading were two key activities for E that she loved, and in cheer she took the traditionally "male" role (being the base for stunts and catching the lighter girls who were thrown up in the air), although this was also fulfilled by other girls, so it didn't seem weird or unusual.

Later on, a few incidents occurred that really showed us how difficult it was to be in this kind of "no man's land". These moments didn't just duplicate some of the difficulties we'd had at home – they made them worse. Two things particularly highlighted the problem. First of all, ahead of a school trip to a local mosque, E was told she had to wear a headscarf to enter because all girls had to wear one. Despite her teachers knowing the situation, they informed E that she needed to respect the religious traditions and wear one. Eventually, when the trip came around, and after some awkward conversations, she just didn't go in, so she avoided the issue.

Then, there was the sports presentation evening at school. Leo was up for quite a few awards. At that point, Bill especially wasn't ready to hear "Leo Telford" read out for all the nominations. We hadn't officially changed Leo's name at school or anywhere else then, either. So, we went for a compromise: L. Leo turned up to the evening with his short hair, trousers and a tie, which was what he wore for school every day. And every time the nominations were read out with the full names of all the other kids, L Telford stood out like a sore thumb. It drew loads more attention to Leo's name than just having Leo up there would have done, and it got more and more painful as the evening went on and all of his nominations were read aloud. Eventually, when he went up to get the awards that he'd won, it stopped being such an issue. People who knew the situation saw Leo as he was, and everyone else just saw a young boy – and probably assumed there was a typo in the presentations deck.

The hardest time at school was probably when Leo went back to school as Leo at the beginning of Year 8. Up to that point, most of the issues we'd come across and dealt with were within the family and were up close and personal. Making the decision to go back to school as Leo, though, was when problems started to be more public, and dealing with them impacted more people.

We realize now that Leo was treated as a special case by his school. He was a special case in the fact that he was the first out transgender child there. But also, some of the arrangements made for him would be hard to duplicate for other trans kids. There isn't a limitless supply of individual toilets, for example.

Now that we're a decade on from when Leo came out, I wonder how that school, and other schools, deal better with trans kids. There needs to be a more "systemized" way of working with them. It does seem weird how so many things are based on gender at school that maybe don't need to be. A bank of individual toilets, all with sinks in them, for example, would take away the problem of single-sex toilets altogether. Dealing with sports and changing rooms obviously takes more thought, but again, there are many reasons a child may not want to change in front of their peers – being trans is just one of them. I don't know the answer and I'm sure schools are having to adapt much more to this stuff. In our experience, because these things were so new at the time, how we were dealt with felt a bit like everyone was finding their way. The main thing was that the school was prepared to try and help, and they did that.

Since I originally wrote this section, sadly, things have not changed for the better. In December 2023, the UK government published the Draft Guidance for Gender-Questioning Children, meant to help schools and colleges better understand trans students, and it's utterly disappointing. Firstly, in the "Overarching Principles" chapter, it states that there has been "a significant increase in the number of children questioning the way they feel about being a boy or a girl, including their physical attributes of sex and the related ways in which they fit into society. This has been linked to gender identity *ideology*, the belief that a person can have a 'gender', whether male ... female ... or 'other', that is different to their biological sex. *This is a contested belief.*"[3] (I added the italics for emphasis.) With that, the entire document undermines the very right of trans people even to exist. It states that being trans is an "ideology", which the Oxford Dictionary defines as a "set of beliefs", rather than a set of facts. Trans people DO exist, whether the UK government wants them to or not! Gender reassignment is even a protected characteristic under the Equality Act 2010! To trans people everywhere, their bodies, and how they feel, think and behave, are not contested – these things are facts.

Getting back to Leo's school experience, though, there were some real bright points, and as there are for so many of us at school, some of those revolved around teachers. One teacher in particular, Miss Lilley – Issy, as we now know her – was Leo's English teacher. She was a massive advocate for the LGBTQ+ community and an absolute lifeline for Leo. At lunchtimes and breaks, Leo would often seek Issy out, and she always offered support. She listened, she understood, and she supported Leo by advocating for him with the other staff and cracking down on negative comments from one pupil in the same English class who was making life difficult for Leo.

Issy was one of a handful of teachers who Leo could and did talk to at school. This group spent a lot of time helping, listening and being supportive, offering advice and being literal shoulders to cry on. Thank you to those teachers, including Issy, Miss Petrovsky and others, who took the time to listen. The fact that there were people there for Leo at this critical time, and in a place where he was having the hardest time, was so important.

The time after Leo came out as Leo at school should, in some ways, have felt like real progress. Leo was accepted not just by his family, but by (most of) his schoolmates, friends and teachers as well. But actually, he had a tough time personally then. For a while, he saw the school counsellor regularly to help him deal with issues that weren't just arising on a day-to-day basis, but some of the issues that I think he had shut away earlier in his transition. Just dealing with his transition was hard enough, but when he spoke to his counsellor, he said how alone he had felt at that time and how we weren't really there for him. He told me a little about it at the time, and I was really upset. I knew he was right, and we hadn't been there when he needed us. He and I have spoken about it again much later, and while we were having some of the conversations we had when writing this book. Of course, I have apologized, and I know Leo has accepted that apology and forgiven me for how I behaved. But I feel that with anything historical like that, there is a rift that will never really be closed, and there will always be a scar.

* * *

Leo

I left my primary school after Year 6 to join a new secondary school the next academic year. It was when I was still in Year 6 that I had come out to my parents. I knew it was too early for me to go back to school as Leo, though I would've been over the moon if that could have been the case. However, my parents just weren't ready. I knew I would sort of have to grin and bear it for as long as it took.

Starting a new school still with my old name while presenting as masculine was a challenge. As soon as I made friends at my new school, I told my close friends that I was trans and I'd prefer if they called me Leo, which they all honoured for the most part. Because my name wasn't Leo on the register, it meant that when talking about me to teachers or to people who didn't know, they would have to refer to me as my old name, as that is what my teachers did for most of the year. On the occasions when this happened, I was always pained, but I was used to being referred to in that way, so I tried my best to ignore it and not take it personally. Over time, the other people and acquaintances in my year caught on, and at the end of Year 7, I was known solely as Leo by my peers.

A key memory I have from that time that really highlights the name problem is my sports awards evening at school. This night often comes up when we, as a family, discuss this period of my transition because it was one of the most uncomfortable but now comical moments. I'd been put forward for some sports awards as, especially in my earlier secondary school years, I represented the school for some sports: dance and cheer. (I did give the cheerleading up in my hyper-masculine phase – we'll get to that later.) Before the evening, my teacher had contacted my parents to see if it was okay to put Leo Telford down as my name. At that point, I was still "Muppet" to Dad, and it was clearly unendurable for him to see me "out there" as Leo, so we compromised on "L Telford". But what we hadn't realized was that the names of all the nominees were projected on a screen for each award – their full names. So, every time, I would come up on stage, the student presenting each award would read the names out, and everyone else's first and last names would be proudly shown on the screen, and then there was just:

L Telford

When I won an award, the guy from Year 11 who was presenting it said, "Well, there's no full name, so I guess the winner is L Telford? So, whoever you are, do you want to come and get your award?" My heart sank hearing that aloud. It was embarrassing, I felt singled out. There was perhaps a crowd of 100–200 people – students, teachers and parents – there. So many students didn't really know me, so I knew they had no idea why I had just an initial representing myself, and I felt awkward and stupid, though I didn't have the greatest choice in the matter. As I walked up, I felt as if all eyes were on me and that everyone was wondering what it was all about. I went up to get my award and spent the rest of the evening hoping I wasn't nominated for anything again.

As we've made clear, things were different then. Even though it was only seven or eight years ago, there was just so little press about transgender people, and my situation still felt new to most of the people I encountered. I was the first out trans kid at our school, and that meant there was no staff training, no experience to draw from, and no guidelines to tackle certain situations or difficulties I was facing. My head of year struggled at the time, and looking back now, I imagine she feels bad about how I was dealt with in my first year at the school. When my teachers were under instruction to refer to me as L, I remember instances when she was angry with me, so she would use my deadname. Whether it was deliberate or not, I can't be sure, but there were moments when it certainly felt that way.

In later years, I came across her in a corridor at school, and I got the impression she was being overly nice, and it felt a bit like she was overcompensating for times when she made the wrong move or was reluctant to take steps in my social transition in the way I desired. Often, trans people – and people of any other minority group – we are wronged out of plain ignorance. I remember one day she called my best friend Sam to her office for a conversation. We were obviously close – best friends – and she decided to ask him, "So, do you feel the same as Leo?"

Sam was confused as to what she meant. He hadn't arranged to talk to her, and she didn't really outline what she wanted to discuss with him before getting straight into it. She tried to make herself clearer.

"You know, do you have the same feelings as Leo? Do you feel like you may want to be a girl?"

Sam realized what she was getting at and explained that she was confusing his sexuality with his gender. He replied, "I'm gay. I'm not trans. I don't want to transition. Just because Leo and I are best friends doesn't mean it's rubbed off on me or anything."

Now it's easy to see how that was an embarrassing moment for everyone involved, but although it was easy for us to laugh about it at the time, it demonstrates the reality of what interactions can be like when people – and teachers especially – aren't educated on LGBTQ+ topics, and how important it is that they are trained on how to talk with and safeguard trans students. I can see how her conversation with Sam came from a place of her as a teacher wanting to offer a student who was potentially in the same position as myself support, but she went about it in very much the wrong way. Luckily Sam wasn't offended, but there are certainly students who would have been when questioned in the same uncomfortable scenario, and her enquiring about a child's gender identity when there was no desire from the student to talk to her about it certainly felt inappropriate.

There were times at school that were made less stressful thanks to thoughtful teachers and staff. Interestingly, I had an easier time in PE, even when a lot of our lessons were still split into boys' and girls' groups. I think to save a lot of heartache and arguments, my teachers let me go in the boys' group without too much of a fuss. This was still before I was officially going by Leo, but they perhaps recognized it would have been harsh and inappropriate to keep me in the girls' group, especially when my female friends publicly referred to me by my male name. I was given sole use of a little room where I'd get changed (I believe it used to be a changing room for staff), as I didn't want to be with the boys because that probably wouldn't have been comfortable for anyone, but of course, I certainly didn't want to be with the girls either. My own room made that easier but was a bit of a one-off solution. It happened because there was a senior PE teacher, Mrs Copley, who was always lovely and accommodating to me. She pulled me aside one day before a lesson, showed me to the changing room and said, "Look, this could just be your room if you'd like." And for the rest of my time at school it was. By the time I was in Years 10 and 11, I would use the men's toilet as I did in public. But it was nice to have my own space to use early on, when I was more nervous and anxious about the social aspect of using a bathroom as a trans man.

One of my big supporters and someone who was always there for me when I was at school was my English teacher Issy, or Miss Lilley, as she was to me then. Now she's a family friend, but she taught me in Years 9 and 10 and made herself visible as an ally to LGBTQ+ students at the school (hers was the only classroom with the "some people are gay/trans, get over it" poster that some readers may have seen before). Due to the fact she is part of the LGBTQ+ community herself, she was one of the only teachers who could truly empathize with some of my experiences, rather than just be sympathetic. As some readers will be aware, there are always memes about how English teachers always befriend the gay kids, and she was a real-life example, which we both found amusing. I spent a lot of time talking with Issy, and she was the person I'd go to when something was troubling me or if I needed a listening ear. At a parents evening when she first met my mum, they joked that they would become friends and go for coffee, just to wind me up, but then they did just that, and to this day she and her partner are close family friends.

Going back a few years to when I was in Years 7–9, we had compulsory German lessons prior to choosing our GCSE subjects. I was fond of my teacher, and during some of my hardest days at school, she was a support I couldn't have done without. I think maybe she just liked me and thought I was a nice kid, but because of how things were at home around that time, and my constant struggle with dysphoria, I was low a lot of the time. Due to this, I would quite often get upset at school and in her lessons, and I would end up spending most of my German lessons in her office. She would just sit and talk to me. Again, I think she knew there was not much she could do, but it was nice to know I had certain teachers to turn to. I know some kids don't have that, and that is really hard because if you're not getting the kind of support you need and desire at home, and it is still inaccessible in the other place you spend most of your time in as a teenager, it can be very lonely.

But as I've said before, not everyone was so kind at the start – and this included my classmates. There was a guy I went to school with who was the head teacher's son. He was in my year and was known to be a bit of a bully, especially when we were in the lower years. He was the ringleader of the big group of boys, and to say we didn't get on for years would be an understatement. In PE lessons he would tell me to go and play with the girls, "where I belonged." He refused to refer to me as Leo for months, making himself the only person in our year group who did so. He would go to impressive lengths to make digs at me at times. As we got older, he calmed down, from Year 9 through to Year 11, we were in English lessons together and would clash quite a lot. We hated each other. Even just to look at him infuriated me because I remembered what he'd been like to me when I was younger, and I hadn't forgiven him as he'd showed no remorse. He behaved like a child constantly, which would piss me off. As I was older and had grown into myself, I didn't take it from him anymore, meaning there were instances we'd get into arguments in class and Issy would have to send one of us out the room to separate us. Eventually, in the middle of Year 11, I switched classes because I couldn't stand being in the same room as him.

At the end of Year 11, on what would become our last day of school (due to the Covid-19 pandemic and lockdown), he came up to me at the end of our business lesson and apologized. He said he knew he'd been a massive dick when we were younger (I had to agree with him), and that he was sorry for it. I was taken aback because although I knew he'd grown up and wasn't the same person anymore, I still didn't expect such a stark admittance of guilt and remorse from him. Though we never became friends, and I haven't heard from him since, I appreciated the gesture, and it was comforting to know people can grow out of such behaviour and ignorance.

For a while, I'd get the occasional question from a classmate and didn't seem to receive too much backlash, mainly just ignorance and misunderstanding. But as time went on people's reactions intensified. By the time I was in my final year at school, I think there was only a handful of students in a school of over 1,200 that didn't know or hadn't heard something about me being trans. At school, telling people was never a choice. It was a decision I was stripped of because it just seemed to spread, and I came to accept the fact because I knew there was little I could do to prevent it from continuing. I would get new Year 7s coming up to 16-year-old me and asking if it was true I "used to be a girl", or if I "had a dick". There were a few occasions when I was in Years 9 and 10 when the word "tranny" was shouted at me down the corridor or whispered under the breath of older boys I had never spoken to before. I'm lucky compared to others that these were the most severe of reactions I've experienced, but for years it felt like a day couldn't go by without being reminded of the fact I am trans and how that made the people around me feel.

Going into Years 9 and 10, I started to make more male friends. I was still best friends with Sam, but I found myself chatting and having a laugh with more boys in my classes than in the first two years at secondary school. These were boys I never would have spoken to because I was intimidated and didn't think they'd be the kind of people I could ever get on with.

In Year 9, I met another one of my best mates, Harry. Categorized as the class clown, he mainly spent lunch and break times flitting between groups in the canteen and on the field, talking to anyone and everyone. We just sort of knew him as the guy that knew everybody. After our first few conversations, he started to come up to my group and me more. In a few classes I was seated next to him, and we found out that we got on well, though this was something our teachers certainly weren't fond of – by Year 11 we spent every lesson being moved away from each other because we were constantly dicking about. He became closer with Sam and me, and we all hung out whenever we could, after school and on weekends. We'd spend our time in town, just hanging out and biking to and from each other's houses and anywhere else we felt like going. Harry quickly became a very good friend. One day I decided to tell him that I was trans. Sam and I got the impression he didn't have any friends that were LGBTQ+. It was fair to say, and he has urged me to mention it when I showed him this section of the book, that he did once have opinions that my friends and I didn't share with him. He was fairly close-minded when he was younger, and he was the first person that I was fond of who I had such differences of opinion with. He wasn't a "lad", so to speak, but he certainly had similarities with that stereotype, hence why

I was apprehensive about coming out to him at first. When I told him, after the initial phase of him not believing me or thinking I was joking, he asked lots of … *interesting* questions. I didn't mind because it was what I was used to, and I wanted him to be educated. The longer we were friends, the more his opinions and viewpoints seemed to shift. Politically, we aren't comparable – Harry has little interest, and I'd categorize myself as a socialist who keeps up with the news as well as I can – but he grew increasingly liberal and open-minded, which all our friends were glad to see. As time went on, we became best mates.

I remember our last day of school in Year 11. A week or so before it happened, we learnt that we were going to be sent home for good without finishing the year in person due to the Covid-19 pandemic. The day was to finish at 1pm, as I suppose they thought we should be at home as soon as possible for safety reasons. So, that day, we all went to the canteen for lunch before we said goodbye. Harry was with me in the queue, and as we got our food, I could see he was hiding his face and shifting away from me as we were talking. We had been saying how surreal and odd it felt that we were finishing the year in March and that we had no idea when we'd see each other again. We'd stopped in the quickly emptying hall, and I asked him if he was okay, putting my hand on his arm to turn him toward me. He hugged me, and as he did so, I could hear his sniffles and I realized he was crying. It was odd seeing Harry cry, as he was never one for expressing much emotion. I patted his back and told him we'd see each other soon. I turned around, as someone else was trying to talk to me, and when I turned back, he was gone. I found my other friends and told them Harry had left and I didn't know where he was. They hadn't yet said goodbye to him, so together we went to look for him. All six of us made our way to the bike shed, where we found Harry alone, unlocking his bike. I think he didn't want to face our goodbye and thought it would be easier to go rather than get more upset. I'd told the others he was upset, so we all went up to him and hugged him. All of us stayed like that for a minute – and a few of us became teary-eyed – and then we decided that we would walk one of our mates home together before the final farewell.

Though I'm at university now and he's at home, to this day, he is one of my best friends. Harry is one of the people who has been so crucial and important in my life, and I don't think he realizes it. I suppose I've never really told him, as we're not the types who have heart-to-hearts often, but he was there for me and allowed me to be myself, despite all our differences, and never made me feel odd or out of place. He treated me just like anyone else, at a time when all I worried about was how different I was to people, especially boys my age. He means the world to me, and I can't thank him enough for being the friend he is.

Chapter 6

GETTING HELP

Gemma

As the months went on after he came out, I could see Leo's feelings weren't going away. They were intensifying and getting steadily worse. We had just moved house, and Leo's room was tucked away upstairs, overlooking the back garden. I would sometimes notice that I hadn't seen him for a little while and go looking for him. I would find him in his room, sitting on his bed with his back against the wall, and he would have been in the same position, just crying, for hours. It was horrible. His room felt so bare and new, and there was no comfort for him. He looked lonely and sad. And he was.

When his periods started, he was inconsolable. He was having to deal with periods, which are hard enough as a teenage girl – not knowing what to expect, the blood, the horrible dragging pain – but he felt even worse. For him, his body was betraying him. In his mind, he was a boy. He felt like a boy. He acted like a boy. It was bad enough being trapped in a girl's body anyway. But that girl's body was maturing, growing and developing in ways that he actively hated. It was really tough, and it was so hard seeing him in so much pain. It was a bit of a turning point for me because when I first read up about being transgender, what I found online seemed to say that it was becoming more usual for kids to question their gender ... but that it was at the onset of puberty that feelings tended to resolve one way or the other. In other words, kids would start to grow up and realize they were happy with their bodies after all, or the opposite – their bodies became a form of physical torture for them that they couldn't escape from. It's called body dysmorphia, and it's not exclusive to trans kids – it's a term that covers anyone who is really unhappy with their body in some way. For trans kids, it can be one of the other key indicators of how they feel about their gender, though.

I wanted to show Leo that I was taking his feelings seriously, and although I had no idea what to do about it, going to see our GP felt like an important step. From the first time that Leo and I went to see him, he was brilliant. (We know now that this is sadly not the case for many trans kids.) We walked down together to his consulting room and sat in the two chairs, with Leo slightly closer to the doctor. I know we were both full of nerves and unsure of what reaction we might get. I could feel my tummy swooping and twisting with anxiety, and I felt on the verge of tears. But our GP was kind and supportive, and he listened to us. I explained why we were there but asked Leo to explain how he felt. I thought it was important for the doctor to hear his precise words and be able to ask the appropriate questions. He did so with sensitivity, and I'm so grateful for how he helped us navigate that first conversation. He listened carefully to Leo, took him seriously and was kind and compassionate. I had tears streaming down my face by that point.

He explained that although coming out as trans was really hard, now was a better time to come out than any previous time in the past. I think he was right in some ways. At least now there is more awareness of what being trans means, more people are encountering trans people and positive steps are being made that mean that coming out as trans is perhaps now that tiny bit easier. (This is in no way to belittle the experience of others coming out as trans now. Just because it's easier doesn't mean it's still not sometimes awful, difficult, heart-breaking and hideous. However,

I live in hope that it's not like that for everyone.) The GP then told us about the Tavistock Centre and said that the practice would support the referral for us. The next GP we saw at our local practice was a lady. We had filled in the paperwork for the Tavistock referral that Mermaids had helped us with, so we took it in for her to look over and sign. Again, she did this happily, and again, it was a positive experience.

Later, when it came time for our doctor to take over the administration of Leo's blocker injections and testosterone, we saw yet another doctor – Dr Prasannan. He was an absolute star. He told us Leo was not his first trans patient, but was only his second. He was interested in the field and asked lots of questions driven by this interest. He has always been positive, good humoured and supportive, and we think he's great. We have really been so lucky with the support from our GPs. The surgery has continued to support Leo as his prescriptions have altered as he's got older. Now, instead of testosterone injections, which started off as every month, then every three weeks, he's on a three-month injection, which is much more convenient, but also saves us having to go backward and forward to the doctor's every other week. The reason for the change was because, throughout the treatment, the Gender Identity Development Service (GIDS), a clinic specialized in children's and adults' gender identity issues, have kept an eye on Leo's blood tests. To start off with, it was necessary to get his testosterone up to a certain level, and that meant having to increase the dose. I would go with him, and he and the doctor would retreat behind the screen for an injection in the top of his bum. The needle was huge, and the testosterone itself is a thick, oily looking liquid, which takes some effort to actually inject in. So, I knew the injections themselves could be quite painful. At the same time, Leo had to have blocker injections to suppress feminine hormones and development. I'm pretty sure he must have felt a bit like a pincushion. Good job he wasn't scared of needles!

On the first visit, our GP also recommended that we visit the local arm of CAMHS, which provides mental health services for kids in the area. It was a good introduction to the experience of family counselling – mainly of how excruciating it could be. I mean that in a good way ... kind of. But we had never been in this type of situation together. (I have – I've had counselling for depression in the past, but we'd never been as a family.) As an adult in therapy, sessions can be excruciating, but at least you only have your own feelings to deal with, however painful they might be. The long pauses while you think of what to say and try to recognize how you actually feel. The shame about some of the feelings that come up. The embarrassment about some of the questions you get asked – *bleurgh* ... I'm sure it can't just be me that feels like that! But as a family, it's worse, I think. You're having to try to deal with your own feelings and be honest, but also moderate what you say so that you don't upset other people or say anything that sounds too blunt or uncaring. It's hard, like splitting yourself in two. Bill finds it even more of a struggle. He's a bit older than me and was brought up by a Geordie dad who would as soon share his feelings as wander round in his pants, and an Italian mother who thinks that men should take responsibility and be men. This does not make for a touchy-feely man.

Our meetings were with two therapists – Phil and Hazel. Phil had worked with another family with a trans kid, so he was seen as having some relevant experience. Hazel worked with kids and usually used art therapy. They were both nice, good people, and I think the main benefit of the sessions for us was that it made us face up to the situation and gave us a safe space to talk, meaning we actually spoke instead of just ignoring things. Although I felt like it was often me talking, Phil and Hazel made sure that everyone got a chance to speak. They asked us all about our opinions on things and to describe how we felt and how things had affected us. There were often tears – usually from me, sometimes from Leo and occasionally from Bill. You'll be unsurprised that Bill was reticent, based on what I've mentioned so far, but he felt that Phil understood him because Phil shared that he had daughters, so he could understand some of what Bill felt by "losing" one. The grief of "losing" a daughter was a huge, real thing. Phil talked about how we were having to "give up" the life we had pictured for our child – the "girly" ways that we had envisaged spending time together, shopping and spa days, wedding plans, what we expected a future for our daughter to be. This was hard to do and come to terms with, but it also showed how much of it was unconscious – we were having to let go of a future that we had planned without even realizing it. But guess what? We didn't have to give up anything. I still go shopping with Leo. One day, he might get married. Nothing has really changed at all. Leo crystallized it for me when he said, "You're not losing a daughter, Mum, I'm still the same person." *D'oh.* Why on earth had I not realized that?

* * *

Leo

My first step toward starting the medical process of transitioning was visiting the GP. Generally, for most trans people in the UK, unless they opt to seek private treatment for the process, your doctor is the first person you turn to. For us, we went there not because we understood it as the "thing to do", but because we didn't know where else to go. I remember that appointment being comprised of apprehension, fear and tears (it sounds a bit like the '80s pop band Tears for Fears, but it was worse). When we were showed into the room, the GP asked, "So, what can I help with?"

The funny thing was, we didn't really know if he could help. When I came out, I didn't know what the Tavistock Centre or CAMHS were, or whether we had even gone to the right place for the initial help we desperately needed. I remember Mum, through tears, trying to explain why we were there, but I could tell she was finding it hard, so I said to the doctor with a wobbly voice:

"I'm transgender."

After that was silence. I heard sniffles coming from Mum shortly after, and as I turned around, I could see her face was streaming with tears. Of course, that triggered the same reaction in me. I've always found it hard to see her or anyone I care about so upset, but something about seeing her so tearful in that moment was particularly hard. What made it worse was that I knew I was the cause of what she was feeling – grief, confusion, pain and hopelessness. I knew what she was feeling because I felt the same. And amongst all of *that*, I still needed help, and I knew I had to hold it together and be strong for us.

After offering us tissues, the doctor began to explain that his first suggestion would be that he put us on the waiting list for CAMHS. Other trans guys I met later also went there as their first sort of step, mainly so they, and sometimes their families, could work on their mental health and work through the often-difficult situations that came with being trans and what that means for a family. Secondly, he told us about Tavistock and Portman, which is the largest and oldest gender clinic in the UK, and where I eventually accessed medical treatment. (In "A Note on Tavistock" on page 136, I discuss my feelings about their "scandal" and how I found it being a patient of theirs at the time it emerged. And how it is essentially a load of *shit*. But like I said, I'll get to that later.)

At the end of our conversation, he referred us to CAMHS as promised and assured us that whilst we were on the waiting list, we could see him again if we felt we needed help or had any questions. I left the office feeling like we'd made a step in the right direction, but I was still hurt and weighed down by what I knew my family and I were yet to go through.

It's crucial to say that we were incredibly lucky with our GP. All trans people have internalized the anxiety that comes with needing to be careful around medical professionals and not knowing whether they've come across trans patients before, because essentially, they are the gatekeepers of our healthcare, and therefore, our mental health too. I've heard of experiences in which trans people have switched GPs and have been denied prescriptions to their ongoing hormone treatment or had to wait far longer than what is recommended or safe to access it. What legitimates these awful scenarios is that, as the University of Cambridge state in their 2023 report on the 2021 GP Patient Survey, there are currently very few guidelines on how GPs should care for trans and non-binary patients.[4]

A few months after our first appointment, we went back to the GP to see if I would be able to go on contraceptive pills to stop having periods. This time, we saw a female GP who was helpful and understood my reasoning – I explained why a 13-year-old boy might want to be on a contraceptive – and she was happy to help.

It took about six or seven weeks before we got to CAMHS. The wait was hard, and my first appointment was an emergency one.

My mum rejected the first appointment offered to us, giving the excuse that my grandparents (who live in Spain) would be staying and that she wanted me to spend time with them. When she told me she'd turned it down, we were in the car, and I remember feeling confused and upset – betrayed, almost. I had been waiting weeks for this, and she knew how desperately I wanted to get there because that meant this was real and I was being taken seriously. I asked her why, but I knew the reason already. She was struggling, so when she was presented with an opportunity to delay a step and conversations she knew she wasn't ready for, she took it. Despite how I felt, I didn't hold it against her.

When we finally went to CAMHS, our sessions were an hour long and most times attended by both my parents and me. There were times my dad didn't come, but this was usually because he was at work and didn't have the flexibility my mum had with her working hours. The sessions were hard but productive because they gave us a dedicated time and space to talk about what was going on. We knew if something had happened that week or there was a time any of us got upset, we would get to reflect on it and gain insight from the counsellors we saw. Sometimes we needed to be guided into having conversations that we knew were difficult to have, and ones we couldn't suitably orchestrate ourselves. We needed someone to oversee how we were all dealing with it and keep track of where my parents were at on their journey to accept my transness. My dad, being an almost stereotypical man in terms of expressing and handling emotions, didn't often verbally contribute to our conversations during the sessions. He would respond when asked questions, but the counsellors would often say things like, "Bill, how do you feel about that?" and he never had much to say. He comes from a family in which communicating, talking about negative feelings or hardships, or being told you were loved weren't the norm. It didn't happen. So, I knew I couldn't blame him for not knowing how or feeling able to navigate and discuss what he was going through. However, there were times he did so. One afternoon, sometime in mid-2017, Mum told me that Dad had sent her an email. At the time, he wasn't communicating at all with us about how he felt, nor did he share the stage he was at in terms of accepting me as Leo. I could only gauge his feelings when there were direct reassurances, for example, when he said it was okay for me to go back to school as Leo in Year 8. Even in those moments, there was no conversation on the matter – if he approved something, then we knew he meant it. In the email to Mum, he expressed his grief for me. As often felt by the parents of trans kids, he felt like he was losing his child, his daughter. I'm not too sure of the content, and that is something he obviously didn't want me to be aware of, but I know how glad and surprised my mum was that he found a way to talk to her about what he was feeling, and grateful that she had a better understanding of his process and feelings.

I knew that having a daughter was one of the happiest days of his life, and for a long time, I carried with me a sense of guilt because I took that away from him. That's not how I look at it now, and I never developed that perspective because of anything he ever said to me, but it took a long time to stop blaming myself for what he went through when I came out. It was out of everyone's control, and there was never doubt in my mind that my parents would prefer a happy, fulfilled child, to one that couldn't guarantee how long they'd be around because they were so unhappy in their body that they might feel they literally couldn't live in it.

Chapter 7

MEETING MERMAIDS

Gemma

My best friend, Teresa, was the person who told me about Mermaids. She knew another trans person, so that's how she had come across the charity. Initially I just filed the information away, as it was still difficult coming to terms with things, and I wasn't sure I could take the next step yet.

But as time wore on, it got really lonely for Leo and for me. I took the plunge and googled Mermaids. Their website is super welcoming and contains loads of helpful information, but in those early days, it just felt like a LOT. I didn't really know where to turn, and it seemed to be geared toward people who knew what they were doing – and I really didn't! They had a parents' group, and in order to join, you had to have a screening call with someone on their team. I was really nervous about it and worried about what I might say – would I get something "wrong"? But when I finally reached out, the lady I spoke to was so lovely. I remember she rang me just as I was parking in Bedford, and so I did the whole call from the dingy car park on Lurke Street (yes, it's really called that).

First of all, I was asked to describe our current situation and why we had contacted Mermaids. I said that I just felt lost – I wasn't sure I was doing or saying the right things, I didn't know where to turn or what to expect. I was worried about how life would be for Leo, what he might have to face in terms of discrimination, bullying, surgery, falling in love. I was catastrophizing. I could only see worries in his future, not joy.

It's funny now, but I was really worried about pronouns back then. It's one of the hardest things to get right early on, and when I speak to people who don't know much about trans issues, it's still one of the things that people get wrong, even when they're trying really hard. They carefully ask me about "your daughter, right, how is she doing?" – thinking that because I used to have a daughter, this is the right descriptor to use. But it's so much simpler – my child identifies as a boy. So, he wants to be called by a boy's name, treated like a boy, and therefore his pronouns have become a boy's pronouns – he/him. The Mermaids lady explained it to me in the same way, and it was like a penny dropping. Even at the stage when I called Leo his new name and got it right almost all the time, when I was talking about him, I would still sometimes get the pronouns wrong. "Ask Leo what she wants for tea." Quite often, this would happen in front of Leo too. *Argh.* He was very forgiving, though, and he could see we were all making the effort. As time goes on, it's amazing how it does start to feel natural, especially when physical aspects of his transition started to make more of an impact. Leo had always dressed as a boy, and even more so after coming out. But he was still slim, fine featured and even with short hair, looked gender ambiguous. Now, of course, he's an absolute tank (I get Mum points for that). He's had years on testosterone, he's worked out regularly, and just before his 19th birthday, he discovered that his biceps were bigger than his dad's, and that he could finally beat his dad in an arm-wrestle. (Bill, who has always been something of an arm-wrestling legend, whose workmates used to take bets on him arm-wrestling other workmen on jobs where he was painting, was slightly disconsolate with the realization that his glory days were behind him.) Anyway, my point is that no one gets Leo's pronouns wrong these days. (Perhaps if you knew what to look for, his small hands and feet might give him away, but his broadness and his beard would make you doubt yourself.)

The phone call with Mermaids was really helpful. I remember shedding a few tears in that dingy car park as, for the first time, I spoke to someone who had been through the same process and really understood how I felt. It was just sheer relief. And then she was able to point me in the right direction about so many things. She told me how to access the parents' group. At that point, it was on Yahoo and was a pain to navigate – now it's on Facebook. She said she would introduce me to another Mermaids mum who lived nearby, so we could meet up. And she also told us about the group meetings that we would be welcome to join. Our nearest one was in Birmingham – still quite a trek for us – but both Leo and I were really keen to go.

On the big day, we caught the train to Birmingham. It was a bright, chilly morning with a gusty wind that made you clutch your jacket closed and hunch your shoulders. I didn't know the city at all, but we had directions for where to go. But what was really nice was that Charlotte, the mum who was running the group that day, sent Izzy, her daughter, who is trans, to come and meet us. This would be the first time either Leo or I had met another trans person. In fact, it was a day of firsts in many ways!

I had Charlotte's number and messaged her to tell her we'd arrived. We exchanged a few more messages trying to find a good place to meet – always harder than it seems when one of you knows the area and the other doesn't! Leo and I then went outside of the station by some steps and saw Izzy looking for us. We knew roughly what she looked like – she was a young woman with long dark hair, slim and of medium height – and she was wearing the same colour coat her mum told us to look for. We breathed sigh of relief. Izzy chatted away while directing us toward the centre, where the meeting was being held. She was clearly unfazed and used to making people feel at ease, which really helped. She was a few years older than Leo, and obviously her experience of transitioning was the opposite to his, but a lot of the feelings were the same. We talked a little bit, and nervously, about our experiences so far.

We arrived at a weird cross between an office and government building – I can't remember where it was exactly, but it had the same kind of vaguely institutional feeling about it that the CAMHS office had. That weird kind of musty smell, walls covered in peeling paint and scuff marks, mismatched furniture that had been picked to be durable, but looked a bit ratty, with sticky wooden arms on the chairs and grey crosshatched fabric on the seats. Through that space, we then walked into a room FULL of trans people! It was the most bizarre experience. It felt scary and validating all at once. There were a mix of kids of all ages, genders and presentations. The small ones, siblings of trans brothers and sisters, went off to play in another room. We took our place in a circle made up of parents and teenagers. There were a couple of older trans boys there, one pre- and one post-top surgery, and I could see Leo's eyes drawn to both of them. Here was the dream, in the flesh. The young lad who had had surgery was wearing Leo's dream top – a plain, white T-shirt. (Leo's wardrobe now contains a ton of these!) No more worrying about wobbly flesh, binders, the wind; no need to wear something patterned, disguising or covered up. Freedom in a T-shirt.

Charlotte welcomed everyone and then especially welcomed the newbies. This consisted of us and a couple called Richard and Dawn, there without their child, who had recently come out as a trans boy – also called Leo, and one year older than Leo. I've never been to an AA meeting, but I imagined that this is kind of what it must feel like. You've got this burden, and you're with a group of people who understand it. You can talk honestly about how you feel and the challenges you've been facing, and the people there get it. And they support you. It was a nervous, emotional, scary, powerful and affirming experience. As Charlotte went round the circle, she got to Dawn and Richard before us. Dawn was about my age with short, spiky dark hair and no make-up. Glasses and sensible shoes.

She looked like she worked in an office and was probably fiercely efficient. Her husband, Richard, in jeans and a sweatshirt, looked a bit confused and uncomfortable. Through tears, Dawn told us about how her daughter had recently come out to them as trans. She said how she felt utterly lost, as if she had failed as a parent in some way, and how she didn't know how to react or what to say. She shared that she was there through desperation. It was as if Dawn had lifted the top off my head and seen into my heart and said all the words I was thinking and feeling. As she spoke, I just felt this huge release and wave of emotion. My hands were shaking, and my heart was racing. And in a matter of minutes, tears were streaming down my face. I did that thing of trying not to sob until the lump in my throat just got too big to swallow. I couldn't sniff enough to hold the tears in – snotty gulps just erupted from me. I'd heard that it's important for people to "speak their truth", but Dawn was speaking mine. When she stopped talking, I just went across the room and hugged her, this woman I had never met. I didn't say anything, and somehow, we just reached for each other. She was shorter than me, and it was awkward, but not awkward at the same time. We both just hugged and cried. We felt exactly the same. Thank God for that. I wasn't alone.

Once we'd sniffed our way to a stop and managed to introduce ourselves, we sat down in a little foursome to talk. Richard and Dawn said it was really helpful for them to be able to talk to (my) Leo and ask questions that they didn't yet feel ready to ask their Leo – and get honest answers. We talked quite a lot about binders, for example. My Leo was already wearing a binder, but their Leo hadn't got one, and they weren't keen. I've written about this in "A Note About Binders" on page 108, so I won't go into it again here. Leo explained exactly why he felt the need to wear one, what it did for him and how it alleviated his feelings of distress about his chest. For me, it was just so amazing to talk to other parents that felt very similar to me and had wrestled with a lot of the same demons. We exchanged numbers and met Dawn and Richard a few times over the next couple of years. Dawn and I even went to an Adam Ant concert together in Birmingham! We visited their house and met Leo and their younger son, and they came to see us a couple of times, too. Leo and Leo talked a lot online and went out together a couple of times. Their Leo went on to have top surgery because he was older than my Leo, and again, it was so useful for us to have insight into their experience. Their Leo was really happy with his result, and it was in part due to this that we chose the same surgeon, Mr Kneeshaw, in Hull, when it was my Leo's turn for his procedure.

Leo and I came away from the meeting feeling so positive. It had been amazing to meet other trans kids and other families and to hear about their journeys. It made us both realize that we weren't doing so badly after all and were coping better than some families had. One poor guy trans guy there was still attending a girls' school. His parents wouldn't recognize his gender identity, so he had to wear a skirt every day and be called by his old name. It was pretty heart-breaking. We also heard about doctors who wouldn't help trans patients and refused to refer them to Tavistock, meaning that, in some cases, families would have to change to a new GP to get the help they desperately needed. Schools were slow to adapt, and in many cases, arrangements weren't being made for trans kids to take care of their needs. But the overwhelming positive for us was that people in the group had gone through a lot of these difficulties and were managing to stay upbeat. Trans kids, despite the prejudice they had been faced with, alongside the physical and social difficulties, were sure about their identities and felt that they had the support of some of their family and friends, and of Mermaids, to help them. We walked back to the train chattering excitedly as the wind blew my hair about so much that I had to keep turning to hear Leo and taking strands out of my mouth to talk to him.

Mermaids was set up in 1995 by parents of gender non-conforming children who wanted to start a helpline for others in the same position, and the brilliant Susie Green had been the organization's CEO since 2016. Susie has a trans daughter, and when she came out, Susie was looking for help, but could find almost nothing in books or online. Even since Leo came out, things are so much better. I think there is much more awareness about transgender issues now, and people know at least what it means, even if they don't know much or "agree" with it. Leo and I were both sad when Mermaids went through a tough time more recently and Susie left. As an organization, the pressure it must be under as a centralized point of focus in the trans debate is immense. Despite having some incredible patrons, who are fantastic role models for trans people – including Hannah Graf, a retired captain in the British Army, and her husband, Jake, a writer, director and filmmaker; the model and author Munroe Bergdorf, and racing driver Charlie Martin – the vitriolic press coverage never seems to stop.

* * *

A NOTE ABOUT BINDERS – GEMMA

Binders are a difficult issue, one which caused Leo and I to have many, many talks, tears and worries. Firstly, I have to say, there are similar issues for trans girls, of course – there are male body parts that are problematic to those in transition. But I can't talk about that here, as neither Leo nor I have any experience with it. If you know a trans girl who has to "tuck" and you want more help with understanding it, a first stop I'd suggest, as with so many other things, would be Mermaids.

So, binders. I understand. Boobs are an issue. They are often in the way and uncomfortable, and so they give rise to a whole host of mixed feelings. For me, when I was pregnant, I felt like my boobs turned into those of a 1950s matron. They were so huge – and not in a good way. I had to wear an unflattering, unboned bra, which shoved them together and gave me a massive crease down the middle. Then, after I had Leo, my boobs had another important role to fill – providing my baby with the milk I'd been storing up. That did not go well at all, so my boobs kind of failed me there. (I know there's lots of support now for women who struggle to breastfeed. I did try quite a lot of it too – help from specialist nurses, friends, NCT people. But I just couldn't get it to work.) What I'm saying I guess is, love 'em or hate 'em, not many of us feel neutral about our boobs. I completely sympathize with how uncomfortable even a small amount of breast tissue made Leo feel. There's a weird wobbly-ness that makes boobs feel like a separate part of you. So, I get it.

Because we were lucky that Leo was able to go on blockers pretty early, which paused his female puberty, Leo was also lucky that he didn't develop too much breast tissue. However, he felt EXTREMELY uncomfortable with what he did have. He constantly walked around with his hand in the bottom of his

T-shirt, holding it away from his body. And clothes were a huge issue. We had to find tops that were heavyweight enough not to cling, that were not see through and that hung okay on his body. Everything he wore had to have some kind of pattern or disguise on it, and layers helped – a shirt over a T-shirt, or a hoodie and a coat. But in summer, it was pretty hellish.

Leo asked about getting a binder fairly early on, having seen trans boys that he followed on YouTube wearing them. There are a couple of companies that made good binders that Leo used a lot: gc2b and Spectrum. There are some things to make sure you do when buying a binder, and the main thing is to properly measure yourself (which, in itself, was a very uncomfortable experience for Leo, so it had to be done from behind and nowhere near a mirror), and make sure you buy the right size. We both know that a lot of trans people size down thinking the flattening effect will be more pronounced, but actually this just makes it super uncomfortable. It's also bad for your ribs. Obviously, as a teenager, you're growing and so is your frame and skeleton, and binders can restrict that growth. The advice is to wear the binder for as little time as you can each day, and never to sleep in it. But again, we know people who literally wore them all the time. After only a few months, Leo started to feel restricted by binders – he would do huge in-breaths because he felt like he wasn't getting enough oxygen in. His ribs and back hurt. But to him, this was all a price worth paying to get a more masculine shape. We tried all sorts of binders, compression vests, cropped bra tops, the works. (Needless to say, this all cost a small fortune too, with many binders coming from the US with extra delivery and import costs.) In the summer, he was boiling having to wear a binder under his clothes, and then clothes that hid the binder. I felt so sad watching him melt in the heat.

At our first Mermaids meeting, we met Richard and Dawn, who, as you'll recall, had a trans son called Leo, just a year older than (my) Leo. They hadn't let him have a binder because they were so worried about them. What was really helpful for them was being able to talk to (my) Leo directly about binders, and see from him how important it was to him and how much more confident it made him feel. They agreed they would let their Leo wear a binder and understood what to watch out for when buying one.

If I thought binders were bad, what Leo tried next was much, much worse: kinesiology tape. This is what you see on runners' legs – the brightly coloured tape designed to hold muscles in place, not tender breast tissue. Leo had again seen online some other trans people who were using tape instead of binders. They talked about it still having the same flattening effect, but it stopped the crushed-ribs feeling and the disrupted breathing. Leo wanted to try it, and he wanted to feel those things too, as well as not being constantly hot. But it was terrible. He taped across his nipples, from the centre of his chest outward, then round the side of his body. It did keep everything still, but changing the tape HURT him. He had huge, red marks that looked, and were, painful. All the blood was being pulled to the surface of the skin when he removed the tape – even if he did it in the shower. It bled and scabbed over. It was bloody awful to see. But there didn't seem to be another alternative – not until surgery, anyway, which was still months and months away. So, what could I do? Not very much. I encouraged Leo to go without tape wherever and whenever he could, and at least tried to get him to give himself some days off from it. I think the fact I practically begged him, often while close to tears, meant he at least took some breaks driven by guilt if nothing else.

Thank God, at the first call we had with Mr Kneeshaw, the surgeon who would go on to do Leo's chest surgery, he told Leo to stop using tape. He said not only would it scar his skin if he continued to use it, but that it might displace tissue and make the operation harder to do or less successful. It was exactly the right thing to say. Leo stopped using tape the next day and I was so thankful.

Leo

The first time I met another trans person (as far as I know) was at a Mermaids meeting that Mum and I went to in Birmingham. It was significant for me because I'd only ever seen other trans people online. The meeting was open to followers of the Mermaids' Facebook page who could make it. Both trans people and their parents were invited. The idea was that those who attended would be happy to provide insight and answer the questions from those who were earlier in their journeys, like my mum and me. When we arrived at the meeting, there were two trans guys: one who'd had top surgery a couple of years before, and one that had just had it. For me, the concept of top surgery felt like a novelty because I'd never come across anyone in real life who had actually had it, and because I was still years away from being of the age to have it, which I couldn't let myself forget or block out. I had only recently become aware of what the operation was, so I was relatively unfamiliar with the process and what it specifically entailed. I remember finding it so exciting and fascinating when one of the guys was talking about his experience of having it, and how happy he was afterwards.

The woman leading the group had a trans daughter herself. Her daughter, Izzy, met us at the station and walked with us to where the meeting was being held. She was shy, but she was friendly, perhaps nine or ten years older than me. When we walked into the room, everyone else was already there, sitting on chairs in a circle, and I'd say there were four or five young trans people there. I don't think there were many parents, apart from a couple, Dawn and Richard, who happened to have a son who had recently come out as trans, also called Leo. (It wasn't at the time, but now, of course, this is quite amusing because I have come to realize all too late how common my name is amongst trans boys. I've yet to learn why, but I can't say I'm too fussed.) We took turns to introduce ourselves, explain who we had come with or if we had come alone, and at what stage in our transition and/or coming-out experience we were. For example, Dawn spoke about the position she was in with her Leo and how much she was struggling to accept him as her son. She explained that she felt as if she was grieving. That really resonated with Mum. When Dawn was finished talking, she began to cry and stopped holding back the tears that had been brewing during her introduction. My mum, who was also in tears because of Dawn's testimony, got up and gave her hug, which they both looked like they needed and felt understood in. The experience meant a great deal to my mum because she hadn't yet met a parent going through the same thing. It was a day of firsts for both of us.

After the group discussion we had in the circle, we broke off, and my mum and I spoke to Dawn and Richard. Richard was curious about binders – what they were and if they were safe – because he explained that his Leo had asked about getting one. At this point, I was binding but hadn't been for long. I told him about the popular company gc2b and how they were probably the best brand of binders at that time, but that they were based in the US, so their products took a while to arrive, etc. Luckily, I knew a fair bit about the safety and guidance of binders because I had to do my own research to convince my mum and dad to let me buy one. I know that such things, especially when someone has no prior knowledge about them, can be daunting, and that naturally parents may be wary. But I could sense that from our conversation, Richard felt assured of the safety and importance of binders to his Leo and trans boys in general, and I was glad that I was able to help him. One thing I have noticed is that, as time has gone on, more people, especially young people, know more about what it means to be trans and certain things trans people do. For example, after I had come out to an ex-partner, we got on to the topics of binding, and as I began to explain what binders were, I discovered she already knew. I was taken aback because I had never encountered a cis person that was already aware of trans-related stuff, especially something like binding. Often, people in the LGBTQ+ community will know about things like "tucking" and binding, likely because of drag and how shows like *RuPaul's Drag Race* have been popularized. Either way, this is a change I welcome because I'm sure it will make trans people's lives a little bit easier in small ways.

After the Mermaids meeting in Birmingham, I felt hopeful. Though I knew the experiences that some of the guys there had gone through were still a way off for me, to meet them and see what the future held reassured me that I would get there too. For both Mum and I, it was an invaluable experience. I knew that meeting, talking with and exchanging worries with Dawn let Mum feel like she wasn't alone in what was happening, and reassured her that what she felt was normal. Though we never attended another group meeting after that, I'm so glad we did – it was exactly what we needed at the time.

Chapter 8

ACCEPTANCE/BECOMING LEO

Leo

I know that, so far, our recounting of our story hasn't been exactly specific in terms of dates, and sometimes even years in which things happened. This is because we never really expected to have to recount it in depth like this, or never thought we'd want to, at least. Most of what we've written about happened eight, nine or ten years ago. Saying this, there is one day I can recall perfectly because I regard it as one of the most important days of my transition – and in fact, of my life. On 22 May 2016, Mum decided that she and I would go shopping in Cambridge. A 45-minute drive away, it was the sort of place we didn't go too often, so it was to be an exciting day already. When I asked what the reason for the occasion was, Mum explained that she wanted us to have a day out together. At that point, we were having the hardest time getting on, and we didn't feel very understood or close to each other, so she thought we should spend some time where it was just us and have some fun.

The other reason, she told me, was because today, she was going to call me Leo. *All day.*

She was taking her *son* out for the day, and she said she would try her hardest to refer to me as such. I was astounded and amazed. It was so unexpected. We hadn't ever spoken about when she might finally start calling me Leo, and every day, all I heard at home was "Muppet", or a sentence that somehow succeeded in referring to me just as a human, as their child, but not as Leo. Not as anyone's son.

I think I replied just with, "Really?" as tears of disbelief and gratitude streamed down my face. It felt as if my heart was about to burst out of my chest. I knew it was just for the day, and that the next morning, I'd return to being a nameless entity because it was still too early for her to commit fully, but the fact Mum could bring herself to make this step told me that it wouldn't be much longer before it all changed. That Sunday was the best Sunday of my life.

I don't even remember what we did particularly. It didn't seem to matter. We could have been stuck on a desert island or told we'd won the lottery – I wouldn't have cared because all I could think about and anticipate was the next time I would hear her address me as Leo. I know at one point, after walking around the shopping centre for a while, we went into Pret A Manger (a personal favourite of mine) for lunch. I picked up a sandwich, handed it to Mum as she was about to pay, and went to find a space upstairs for us to sit. As I walked up the stairs, not taking notice of the conversation she was having with the cashier before, I heard her say something to the effect of, "That's for my son." That was the first ever time I had been called that. Her *son*. I smiled so hard as I walked up the stairs that people passing must have wondered what was wrong with me.

When we sat down together, we chatted for a while and ate our food. When we'd finished, Mum was on her phone for a while. I assumed she was just replying to an email or something as she did often and didn't take much notice. After a few more minutes, as I was beginning to wonder if she was, in fact, typing an essay, she handed me the phone and asked me what I thought of *this*. On the screen was a silver ring on a jeweller's website. I didn't understand what and why she was showing it to me. I said, "It's nice, who's it for?"

"It's for you" she replied. She took the phone back and scrolled down the page a tad. She handed it back to me, and in a box where you could write a custom message to be engraved on the inside of the ring, I read the following words:

"22.05.16 Love you, Leo."

She explained that she wanted me to have something to remember this day by. After I received the ring, I wore it ring every day. It meant the world to me. Unfortunately, though it was so precious, I somehow lost the ring about three years ago. It was so important to me in those first few years after I'd come out because it was a constant reminder and reassurance that I was accepted and loved as myself. As I've got older, and the longer I've lived as Leo, the less and less I need such a thing to tell me what I already know. Though it was such a shame I lost it, my acceptance now is around me every day.

Before that day in Cambridge, my mum went on a work trip to the US for two weeks. Though at this point I was a teenager, it felt odd that she would be away from home for so long because she'd never done that before. At that point, we were very much *between* everything still. It was still "Muppet" from Dad and pronoun avoidance from Mum and answering to different names from different people, and ultimately, everyone still felt lost. Whilst she was away, Luca, Dad and I would videocall her every few days when we could find the time (because of the time difference), but it was odd without her being there. When she got back, we were all so glad to see her, and once she'd settled back in to being at home, I offered to help her unpack. As we were upstairs folding clothes and putting her things away, she was telling me about what she'd been up to. For a moment, there was a break in conversation, and she stopped still, turned to me and told me, "I get it now." I asked what she meant, though, of course, there was a burning, hopeful inkling that I knew what she was getting at. She replied, "I know that you're my son."

Talk about a choker. I didn't know what to say. I flooded with tears and relief and hugged her. I didn't need to say a thing, and we both knew that.

Shortly after these two moments between Mum and I, slowly but surely, she began to call me Leo. For good. There were hiccups and wrong pronouns left, right and centre at first, but she was a parent having to re-learn how to address her child, so of course that was the case. It was a little sting every time she got it wrong, but a little sting compared to not being her son was nothing. Writing this book has been the most I've thought about these moments of my transition in years. Looking back, it feels alien to recount the time when my parents couldn't and didn't yet accept me as their son.

When I started this process, it didn't occur to me to write about how I accepted myself. It never crossed my mind because for so long as a teenager, I subconsciously didn't think I deserved the privilege to contemplate or come to terms with how I felt about being trans. I was so concerned and invested in my parents' process of accepting me that I didn't stop to let myself feel or think too deeply about self-acceptance. For a long time, I had a vague sense of resentment about my identity. I would wish it wasn't the case, pray – though I am not and never have been religious – that I would wake up the next morning as a cisgender boy and be allowed to just get on with my life. I hated how hard it made everything: my relationship with my body, my school life, my appearance, romantic relationships, intimacy. The burden felt never-ending. Then, there were sometimes moments, not as often as there should have been, in which I would feel overwhelmed with a sense of pride about being trans and regret all the time I had spent trying to cover it up.

Coming to terms with my sexuality – I'm bisexual – and how this intersected with my transness was something I struggled with mentally, sometimes more than being trans itself. I believe it came from the notion I had created and internalized of thinking that being bi and trans was just "too much"; that I was making myself so hard to accept and understand; that it might seem to others like I just wanted these labels to "fit in" or make myself appear as something I'm not. I had internalized these horrible thoughts and reactions, but as I've got older, I've learnt to let them go. However, I am only young, and I am only human, so of course there are times when I adjust things or limit the knowledge I share about myself in the presence of others to make what I'm sharing more digestible, but I think is something everyone does at times. And we shouldn't feel the need to, but to a degree, it's just the way it is.

But acceptance is a never-ending process as a trans person. In every walk of life or new relationship, we risk not being accepted for who we are. We know that sometimes being visible as trans means endangering ourselves and making us vulnerable, in some cases to hostile or violent reactions. After someone transitions (to the extent they desire), everything doesn't just stop. Just because I now am legally identified as and appear male, that doesn't mean I am no longer trans. Our transness is forever with us and cannot be forgotten. There is a duality to this notion that can make us (trans people) feel conflicted. In one sense, it can feel like an inescapable burden because, though now we may live happily in our new identities, we know that we can never disconnect from our past – it is something we will carry around for the rest of our lives. But the other side of this is the everlasting impact being trans has on a person – and not in the gloomy sense I've already discussed. Instead, we have the privilege of knowing we have gone through emotional, mental and sometimes physical turmoil to reach the place we knew we needed to be, and we lived to get there. We get to carry our stories and that knowledge with pride, and always have a reminder of how we have fought through our difficulties to be who we are today. For me, being trans means being strong and defiant, unwavering in one's ability to achieve fulfilment. So, when people ask me, do I ever wish I wasn't trans, I will always proudly reply, 'No.'

Chapter 9

TAVISTOCK

Gemma

We had a nine-month wait between our referral from the GP to our first Tavistock appointment. One day, a letter arrived for the "Parents or Guardians of Leo Telford". It looked official, and we suspected it must be from the Tavistock. Leo was elated. He saw this as "the beginning". Even though he was now Leo at school, this appointment marked the first stage in his official transition, as he saw it. The appointment came through for 31 January 2017 – Luca's birthday. Luca was still young enough (nine years old) for his birthdays to be a really big deal, and it was hard telling him that Leo and I wouldn't be at home when he got back from school because we'd be in London, and only the two of us could go. So, we did Luca's presents before school, and he had some friends round for a birthday dinner afterwards. As I've mentioned before, even when he was really small, Luca was very accepting of Leo's transition, so he knew what a big deal this appointment was.

We caught the train to London in plenty of time, and then got on the Tube to St John's Wood. We still had enough time to spare, but then Apple Maps did its usual thing of telling us to go one way and then the other, and we found ourselves crossing and re-crossing the busy road outside the Tube station, trying to work out which way to go. We eventually figured it out, and the clinic was only a ten-minute walk away. We arrived and still had a few moments to spare, so once we'd worked out where the entrance was, we sat outside on the wall and took the inevitable commemorative photos. It's fair to say that Leo was positively beaming. The photos show a young boy with as a big a smile on his face as it's possible to have, squinting in the sunshine.

Once we were inside the Tavistock, the complexity continued as we tried to navigate the corridors and floors to find the right waiting area. We could tell instantly when we'd arrived in the right place, as packed into the tiny room were a number of other kids and parents, all displaying a variety of gender-neutral clothing and the same semi-terrified expressions that I'm sure we had on our faces too. The room had a tiny white coffee table in the middle with some random magazines, and about six inches of space either side before you hit someone's legs. It was impossible not to look around at the other parents, and you couldn't just divert your eyes and pretend you were in a different place – we were all too packed in. Some of the parents seemed keen to swap knowing smiles with me and others, and some kept to themselves. Conversations in rooms like that are always weird, as the room is so quiet, and you know that basically anything you say is said to the whole room.

On arriving, you had to ring a bell next to a glass window, and then someone came along, opened the window, checked your name and told you to wait. After all our visits, I can't say that it was a great experience waiting. The whole sliding glass window thing felt a bit weird, like we all had a dirty secret and needed to talk quietly. But maybe that's just me. I'm not good with hospitals and medical-type places in general – to me they feel really institutionalized and impersonal.

We waited as other families were collected by their therapists one by one, and we passed the time by trying to work out if we would have liked those therapists for ourselves or not. Most looked pretty friendly, and everyone in the room appeared to be familiar with their therapists, so it seemed that it was only us there for the first time.

After a while, two ladies came to collect us. I'll call them Nadine and Sophia. Nadine was a bold, bright and confident young Black woman with an open smile and a firm handshake. Sophia was a quieter, more softly spoken, bespectacled and studious-looking white woman, with an end-of-the-fingers handshake, the sort I hate, unfortunately. I tried not to hold it against her, but I automatically felt more drawn to Nadine. We followed them down a corridor with the cheap blue carpet loved by institutions across the country and into a tiny room. It had low armchairs, a boiling old-school ridged radiator and a round wooden table in the middle with a box of tissues front and centre, as found in the offices of counsellors everywhere. I always hate the symbolism of those tissues. On one hand, I guess it's saying openly that emotion is okay here, and it is expected. But on the other, it seems to be a challenge – you know you're going to need me sooner or later. And yes, I almost always did. Bloody tissues.

The first meeting was very much a "get to know you" session. We both talked in turn about the process and our experiences to date in getting to the appointment, how we felt about it and what we could expect. What we could expect turned out to be a pretty lengthy process, wherein the therapists would try to understand how Leo was feeling and help him explore his emotions. It was made very clear to us that this process had to completed before there would be any access to medical treatment. We already knew a bit at this stage about hormone blockers and testosterone, and Leo knew that he wanted to go onto blockers as soon as possible. The therapists were very keen to point out that these would be some distance away, that there was a lot of "thinking" to do before then, and only at the end of this initial period would they write a report and recommendations. And they expected that to be months away, maybe even a year. It felt a bit dispiriting.

I know there has been tons of negative coverage and criticism of the Tavistock, to the point that its closure has been announced and it is due to be replaced with alternative facilities. Some of the criticism has suggested that therapists in some way "pushed" children into a diagnosis of being transgender and having body dysmorphia. Some cases have centred around the fact that, very occasionally, children who have taken sex hormones have later on changed their minds and wanted to de-transition. I can only speak about our experience, but I will say that this was never, ever the case for us – it was quite the opposite, actually. Instead of Leo being encouraged to identify as trans, we felt like his thinking was questioned at every level. We never felt like he was being judged, but only that the therapists wanted to be as sure as they could be – and for Leo to be as sure as he could be – that the path he was choosing was the right one. They accepted that, at any point, he had choices ahead of him – he might explore his gender, sexuality or presentation in any way he felt he wanted to and come to any conclusion, and it was all okay. Over the following months, we had many, many discussions about really tough topics – frequently reducing both Leo and me to tears. But I never felt that these were undertaken with anything except Leo's best interests at heart.

When people say that transitioning gender is "too easy" – and especially with some of the criticism that was aimed at the Tavistock that they were somehow "encouraging" kids to identify as transgender in the rush to give them hormones – all I can say is, I have no idea who those people spoke to. Certainly, our experience could not have been more different. Leo was challenged in his thinking at every visit – we all were. Sometimes it felt less like a challenge and more like having to prove ourselves. Conversations could be extremely direct and often felt almost brutal. We were asked to consider every question from every angle: Why did Leo feel as he did? What was behind those feelings? How, as parents, did we feel about Leo and his feelings? What if his feelings changed – what then? We were asked to consider all sorts of viewpoints, and then we had to explore why we thought blockers and testosterone were the right thing – what if they weren't? What effects were we expecting? On and an on it went for months and months. Leo was asked about his future fertility – what if, at some point in the future, he wanted his own children? The therapists explained that the effect on future fertility was not really known, so we should consider the worst-case scenario – that Leo would effectively become infertile.

Then there was a horrible discussion about whether or not Leo wanted to freeze his eggs before starting any hormone treatment. We duly went away and researched what this would involve: basically, they would boost Leo's oestrogen levels, and then harvest and store his eggs. He didn't want this – not just because it sounded like a pretty grim process – but because, as he explained it, not being able to fertilize an egg in the same way as a cis man would make him feel like a "failure" in some way. As you can probably imagine, it's incredibly difficult to have these conversations with your teenager. They didn't affect how he felt about himself – he was a boy. But they could have affected things that he might want at some time in the future, and honestly, I don't know how kids are supposed to know all that stuff. For me, when I was married for the first time at 21, I was absolutely adamant that I never wanted to have kids. It was only when I re-married at 30 that I changed my mind! In my 20s, I'd actually considered being sterilized – that's how sure I was that I would never want kids. (As I said before, I only decided against it after a conversation with my mum, who advised me not to "in case one day things change".) I explained this to the therapists and said I didn't see how they could expect Leo to see into the future any more than I'd been able to as a young married woman.

Sometimes on our Tavistock appointments, we were joined by Bill and a couple of times by Luca as well. The team were keen to understand and see more of the family dynamics, which I also understood. Sometimes Leo went off with Nadine, and Bill and I stayed in the room with Sophia while she did her best to dig into our feelings. Luca actually brought some light relief to the sessions he attended, asking lots of questions, which were inevitably met with the response, "Well, what do you think, Luca?" Luckily, he's never been backward in coming forward, so he was normally happy to tell them both what he thought. And Nadine and Sophia were impressed with his questions and his answers.

After over a year of regular visits, we finally got the longed-for report that would determine the next steps in Leo's transition process. This was the considered view of our therapists, approved by the internal team. We got the report when Leo was 14, and to be honest, it was disappointing. Although they praised Leo for his maturity, thinking and consideration of all the options, and although they knew we were behind his decision to request blockers as soon as possible, they recommended that we wait another year before starting them, because to do so at this stage would represent "early intervention", which they were keen to avoid. But why would we wait? Puberty was already starting to change Leo in ways he absolutely hated, and which would be irreversible. He had started his periods, and they were awful. He was already taking medication to stop them – the contraceptive pill. So, it just seemed crazy to wait to take another form of medication that would stop them. We knew that blockers would press pause on Leo's puberty. They were originally developed for precocious puberty – girls who started their periods too young would take them to give their bodies time to adapt and grow up. We were told that these girls would resume a normal puberty when they stopped taking the blockers. The problem was that the drugs had not been specifically approved to stop puberty in transgender children. To me, this seemed like splitting hairs. They were approved and safe for young girls to use to stop their periods and halt their puberty. Leo was still biologically a girl. He wanted to stop his periods and his female puberty – what was the difference?

Tavistock agreed that if, as parents, we wanted Leo to be able to start blockers, they would allow it, making it very clear that this was our decision, not theirs, and that we were going against their recommendation. Again, I understand why perhaps this all felt necessary to them, but to us, the dangers of Leo's body becoming more developed and feminine seemed a much bigger risk. We already knew he was thinking about top surgery to remove the small breasts that were developing. We didn't want his body to develop a more feminine shape that would be almost impossible to change later. I still struggle with this thinking from the gender-critical people out there who think that putting kids on blockers is somehow harming them. They are completely reversible (otherwise, why would they be given to very young girls in the first place?). To me, it makes absolute sense that, if you give transgender kids blockers when they are younger, it allows them some space to be in charge of what happens next to their bodies. It can hopefully reduce the need for more extensive surgery later, and can address many of the issues caused by body dysmorphia and seeing their bodies "betray" them (this is how Leo saw it) by changing them into something and someone they are not.

So, eventually, it was agreed that Leo would receive a prescription for blockers and would get his first injection at University College London Hospitals (UCLH).

Toward the end of our time with Tavistock, we started working with a new therapist – I'll call her Laura. We did see her in person a few times before the Covid-19 pandemic, and after that, it was all online. Laura was very different to our previous therapists, and perhaps it was because Leo had been living by himself for some time and had started to really grow up and mature, but she was so lovely, and I think just what we both needed by then. She was a small, compact lady with snuggly looking jumpers, cords and sensible shoes; short, feathery hair; soft blue eyes and a face full of character. She was understanding, helpful and warm. By that time, Leo was already on testosterone, and Laura was really just checking in with us to make sure he was okay and his treatment was on track, and then providing a link between the Gender Identity

Development Service (GIDS) and UCLH, who would take over Leo's care once he was an adult.

There was another weird in-between period when Leo was 17 and 18, again caused by the pressure on health services in the UK. As Leo had been a Tavistock patient, his care would automatically be transferred away from GIDS, which only looked after children. We could select which adult clinic looked after him. Most people chose Charing Cross (now known as Gender Identity Clinic, London), and so did we. However, despite the fact that Leo was deemed a "priority" case because he'd come straight from Tavistock, there was still the inevitable waiting list. At that time, it was still over two years long, and our meetings with Laura carried on for much of that time. Eventually, Leo had his first call with Charing Cross, and he is still being cared for by them. In fact, again, it's really more just a check-in, request for blood test to check his levels and shared care with Leo's GP.

* * *

Leo

The next step in getting help was to start my process at Tavistock. By the time I received a letter about my first appointment, I had been on the waiting list for seven months. Seven months felt like a lifetime for me. I thought about my first appointment every day. It loomed over me constantly. I was so excited for it because I knew this was the first *real* step, as it would be the place where I would finally begin my medical transition. Trans people in the UK, and their friends and relatives, will know how short the wait I experienced was, compared to the horrifyingly long waiting periods trans kids are subjected to now. Years-long waiting lists are the reality for those wishing to transition at the time of writing this book. I know of trans people who went on the waiting list with the Tavistock at 14 or 15 years old and began their transitions at age 18 in adult services, meaning that they were never seen in all the years they waited for an appointment with the children's clinic. Needless to say, such a wait can have a worrying effect on some young trans people and can be dangerous. Already, suicide and rates of poor mental health among trans kids are upsettingly high, but when transitioning seems so unachievable –I'm sure it's almost mystical to some – how can this be expected to improve when medical intervention is, for many, *the* thing they need? Whilst some are lucky to be seeing CAMHS, counselling is not the type of support that can change lives like transitioning could.

It's important to make clear that I am not talking about all trans people when I refer to this burning desire to transition. Transitioning, and the extent to which people do so, varies massively within the trans community across the world. Those who identify as trans may never feel the need to physically alter themselves – simply being recognized as something other than what they were identified as at birth is enough. Some will be on hormones but never desire surgery, or they may wish to only have specific surgeries. For example, among trans men, it is common to be on hormone treatment and have top surgery – a masculinizing type of double mastectomy – but at the same time, there's much less interest in bottom surgery, which probably needs little explanation! The reasons for people's reluctance for certain medical intervention also varies greatly and is dependent on personal and economic factors. For some, it could be that they feel they would not be satisfied with the standard of results and therefore delay this specific stage in their transition. Then, there are those who aren't lucky enough to have nationalized healthcare, or they live in places where gender-affirming surgeries aren't available for free, so they simply can't afford an operation that could cost them thousands. For context, at the time of writing this book, top surgery typically costs many thousands of dollars in the US, whereas in the UK, we paid just under £8,000.

I was 14 when I had my first appointment at Tavistock on 31 January 2017. Unfortunately, it fell on my younger brother's birthday, but considering the context and length of time we had waited for this moment, he understood that my mum and I weren't able to be there for a few hours in the day, and we all went to Pizza Express the same night to celebrate instead. I remember the feeling when Mum said there was a letter addressed to me in the post. At the time, considering my age, there weren't many reasons why I'd receive letters, so my first thought was that it could be from Tavistock. As I went to retrieve it, I attempted to calm myself down and prepare for disappointment – that way, if I was wrong, it wouldn't matter so much. I went into the living room and opened it. The first line I read was an appointment date, then my eyes darted to the top of the page, and I read the words "The Tavistock and Portman NHS Foundation Trust". My eyes welled up.

The slot we were given was around lunchtime, so late that morning, Mum and I set off to London, which luckily is only an hour's train journey away from Bedford. The whole day, I had that sort of squeezing feeling I get in my chest when I'm nervous and excited and anticipating something I've been thinking about for so long. It's funny because really the sessions themselves are nothing to be excited about, as they were often challenging, and made me think about and discuss things that could be tricky to face and tackle. They certainly weren't without tears at times. Nevertheless, it felt like the start of an unexpected journey (call me Bilbo Baggins) that I couldn't wait for.

When we arrived in the building, a short walk from St John's Wood station, we climbed a few flights of stairs and entered a tiny waiting room. It had seats and a table of magazines to keep our anxious selves busy (although we were too nervous to read), and a glass barrier at the front desk. We went over, said who we were and when our appointment was, and the receptionist instructed us to sit down until we were fetched by our clinicians.

I don't remember my first appointment all too well, in honesty. I wish I did, but the reason I don't is most likely because it wasn't particularly memorable in content. We discussed my history, how long I'd been out, and how I had found the process so far. It was a chance for us to get know each other and for them to understand the context of my journey. In most of the sessions we attended, Mum and I (and sometimes Dad too) would start in the same room, where we'd have a short chat about how things had been recently, and then we'd split off into separate rooms. We always spent the session with the same clinicians – me with a lady I'll call Nadine, and Mum and Dad with a woman I'll call Sophia. We all were fond of them both, which certainly made it easier to talk to them about such troubling and personal experiences.

In my discussions with Nadine, I would often get upset to varying degrees – not because she made me feel this way, but because the things she would get me to analyse about myself or discuss were often heavy and large in scale of importance. For example, when considering hormone therapy, I had to decide whether I wished to freeze my eggs. To this day, I am regularly consulted about this when in meetings with my doctors, but if I was to decide to do it, before testosterone (T) would have been the best time for it in terms of fertility. That's because one of the risks or side effects of being on T was that I would likely become infertile. This is not always the case, and I'm sure some of you will have come across news stories of older transgender men who have carried babies before, but it is generally understood that you become less fertile the longer you undergo hormone replacement therapy (HRT), which is literally what taking testosterone does – replace the hormones in your system. This means that if I had been on T for ten years and decided to have eggs harvested so my partner and I could have a biological child together, the eggs would probably not be viable. Having to consider a decision of such overwhelming importance when I was 14 and 15 was daunting and scary, to put it mildly. Some of the questions from that session were things like, "What if you were in a relationship with somebody in the future and they wanted kids, and they wanted you to have a biological child?" It was challenging to think about so many "what ifs". At the time, I remember feeling dysphoric about the idea of using a sperm donor if I were to have children with a woman. I hated the idea of another (cis) man providing what I can't. I don't think the same way about such things now – and have felt for a while that if I was to want children in my future, I would prefer to adopt – but it just shows how the ways you think about things can change over time.

Another one of the topics I would discuss with my clinicians in sessions at Tavistock was how I felt a real pressure and desire to be hyper-masculine. Because I was a young trans guy, I was visibly behind all the boys in my year in terms of physical development. This was something I felt dysphoric about and struggled with until I was on T for a few years. I fought for years with the desire to be as typically "manly" as I could, to experience validation from others around me, but I think also to feel validated within myself. I had a deep-rooted notion that the more masculine and "straightforward"' a trans person I was, the easier my identity would be for people to comprehend, accept and respect. The more valid I would be. I think for a lot of young adult males generally, these are typical issues. It's no secret how young men often fight to express emotion and deal with things through anger and confrontation, rather than through sensitivity, vulnerability about their emotions and communication. Despite the fact that this is less of the norm now, there is still always a pressure to "just be a man about it". During this period, I internalized such notions deeply. I literally wouldn't sit in certain ways because I thought I looked feminine. I wouldn't listen to music that I thought could be deemed feminine. I really ignored my attraction to boys because I thought that feminized me, too. I thought that it was emasculating. These are all things I've come to accept as utter horseshit, of course, because I've grown up and become so much more comfortable in myself and my masculinity. But those are the things I really, really struggled with, and it affected me day to day for a long time.

My assessment period at the Tavistock took the best part of a year. They use the phrase "assessment period" to refer to the time it takes them to get to know an individual and gather evidence to decide if the intervention they wish to access is right for them. In my case, due to my age, when I had my first appointment at the clinic, I was too young to legally start HRT, so I wanted to go on hormone blockers. Hormone blockers have been used previously/ are still prescribed to young girls who start menstruating at an age deemed too early, but it is understood that they have also been used to treat transgender children since the 1990s. They are taken as an injection. The injection suppressed my oestrogen to prevent me from experiencing female puberty further. It was important for me to access these injections because, as I'm sure you realize by now, going through the puberty associated with your sex assigned at birth is incredibly difficult and harming for a trans person. I couldn't face feeling like I was becoming a woman, and having to go through female puberty to the full extent would have been detrimental for me personally – and this is the way many trans children think about it. Due to my age, Tavistock didn't recommend that I begin hormone blocker treatment when their report finally came out, which happened about a year after I started seeing them. As a rule, they didn't tend to recommend it to individuals under the age of 16, and I was 15 at the time. But their recommendation, or lack thereof, doesn't stop a patient from accessing the treatment. They explained that although this was their verdict, it wasn't due to anything personal about me or my gender dysphoria/"incongruence", as it is now called, and that if my parents consented, I would still be able to start treatment. And that is just what we did.

At age 16, I begun taking testosterone. As I'm sure is clear, this was always something I knew I would do, as I did not feel I would be able to live freely and happily if I could not medically transition. At the time of writing this book, I have now been on T for six years. This means that I have essentially gone through what some medical professionals refer to as a "second puberty". Within the first few months of taking T, my voice broke and was croaky, and then it dropped. I started to grow more body hair and facial hair (very slowly at first though – much to 16-year-old Leo's disappointment), and I experienced fat redistribution and better progress at the gym. Every new change, no matter how small or mundane, meant the world to me. To get to watch myself become more masculine in such physical ways was the most fulfilling and thrilling thing in the world to me.

Now, I sometimes take for granted that I'm a 20-year-old man with a beard and a hairy chest because I've been this way for so long now, but without hormone therapy, this wouldn't be the case. Being on T and having top surgery have been the most important and life-changing events for me. The longer I've been on T, the happier I've become. To think that I've become the man I am today, in place of the a nervous, depressed and dysphoria-ridden trans boy I was, is unexplainable. I am so lucky and privileged to have been able to access medical intervention as, for various reasons, this is unachievable and painfully difficult to do for so many trans people globally.

I was under Tavistock's care from the age of 14 until I was 20, at which point I was discharged. Usually, you are discharged when you become an adult and are handed over to what is referred to as "adult services". Due to adult services being overwhelmed, and because of the increase in trans people in the UK being referred to Tavistock over the last few years, I had to stay in the care of Tavistock until I could be seen by adult services. There was no need for me to have regular appointments with a clinician during this period, as at that stage, I was with them as a formality, but my medical transition continued to be overseen and reviewed at regular intervals by the endocrine team at University College London Hospital (UCLH).

A NOTE ABOUT TAVISTOCK – LEO

Every discussion I had with clinicians at Tavistock was a far cry from the way they are portrayed in the press, where they were said to have encouraged children to transition. These unsubstantiated and inflammatory claims are designed to fuel the moral panic that poisons the discourse around trans people – children and young adults specifically – and our rights.

The Gender Identity Development Service (GIDS) at the Tavistock and Portman NHS Foundation Trust opened 35 years ago. It was one of the only gender identity services in the UK. There were only eight of them in total, so this one was a crucial and important place for thousands of trans kids and young adults. For many, it was where they first received recognition and support for their mental health and gender dysphoria, where their needs were considered and attended to, and for some, it was where they began their medical transition.

The *Bell v Tavistock* case in 2020 was arguably where the controversy around the clinic began to build. For those who aren't familiar, Keira Bell is an ex-patient of Tavistock who entered the service at age 16, went on puberty blockers and had top surgery, and then realized in her early 20s that it was not the right path for her. She later sued the clinic, claiming that Tavistock "failed to protect young patients who sought its services", and instead of providing "careful individualized treatment," conducted "uncontrolled experiments" on its young patients,[5] thereby attributing some level of blame to them for her decision to detransition. The initial impact of the case was devasting for the thousands of trans and gender-questioning young people on the waiting list, as it was ruled by the High Court that any individual under the age of 16 is unlikely to be able to consent to hormone blocker treatment.[6] (This has since been overturned due to Tavistock's appeal.) Bell's detransition was a personal choice. In the UK, one survey showed that only 0.47 per cent of patients had transition-related regrets, and an even smaller percentage of that group made steps to detransition. It's also important to note that reasons for detransition are not all fuelled by regret. Thirty-six per cent of those surveyed by Gender GP listed "pressure from parents" as their motivation, with "harassment and discrimination" also being one of the most influential factors (31 per cent).[7]

Of course, every case and clinician is different within such a large and specialized service like Tavistock, and no can know for certain whether Bell's treatment *was* rushed, or why she felt that Tavistock did not fulfil their duty of care. However, the lack of other cases like hers against the clinic points to how rare such misfortunes are. It isn't without merit to say that part of the reason the case gained so much media attention and created such controversy around Tavistock was due to the transphobic and ignorant nature of the British media. I have friends who, by 2020, had already been on the waiting lists for years, hoping to begin hormone blockers after their assessment period, who had to find out they would have to wait until age 16 to even be considered, so their referrals were paused. The real effect here was that such individuals could not start medically transitioning until they reached adult services at 18 because they spent the entirety of their time with GIDS on the waiting list. This meant, among other detrimental side effects, that they had to experience a full puberty. Whilst I'm sure there are people that feel the Bell case has "protected" younger trans/gender-questioning children, the detrimental impact it had on the lives, safety and mental health of thousands of other trans people was far greater. It is only fair of me to say that what I've discussed here are views of my own, but to say it is purely a matter of opinion feels limiting, and I know I echo the views of many others who have experienced this.

When an independent person decides to take a medical step at the clinic, guided by the advice and resources provided to them in a careful and structured process, then ultimately what they choose to do is their choice (and that of their parents). Tavistock knows that if a person changes their mind about an aspect of their transition, it can come back to them, as happened with Keira Bell. This is why they were so rigorous and thorough in sessions and discussions with their patients when talking through what certain steps will mean for them and their future. I know that, for me, I was challenged at every turn and made to think about some really, really hard stuff, especially considering how young I was at the time. The clinicians know that they have a responsibility, despite how tricky and uncomfortable some conversations are, to fully assess and make their patients aware of all possible implications and meanings of the decisions they make there.

A 2023 article by the *Guardian* about GIDS highlighted the testimony and nature of experiences of other trans people in the service, and why those that spoke to the paper were "fearful" to "lose a space to explore their gender identity". One testimony by 21-year-old Tyler describes how GIDS was a "lifeline" for him, a place in which he felt that he was treated with "nothing but respect".[8]

A lot of the sessions I had with my clinicians were spent discussing what my medical and general hopes for the future were. When I expressed desire for a certain change, such as undergoing top surgery or beginning testosterone, I was questioned about it. At first, the answers seemed obvious, but they wanted me to understand what within myself drove my desire for physical intervention, and what the outcome would be if it didn't happen. Could I live without it? Such things were tough to think about and assess, but without going through such processes, I can't guarantee that my clinicians and I would have been as confident as we were in my diagnosis of gender incongruence, my transness, and my desire to medically transition. Hearing that clinicians were accused of "skipping over" or not questioning patients to the best of their ability infuriates me because such claims are worlds away from my experience. I know a lot of trans people have found this endless negative reporting upsetting and distressing. And I think the way certain conversations around the clinic have been conducted were an attempt to damage something that's so vital for the (young) trans community in England. And unfortunately, they succeeded.

The "contentious" nature of the Tavistock is something that has been constructed. The impact one person's experience has had on the thousands of others was devastating. Many people, myself included, were dumbfounded by the outcome, and how it ultimately set back transgender rights in the UK. Never in my time with the clinic did I *ever* feel pressured, neglected, overlooked, misunderstood or rushed into choices that were not my own. The sense of relief I felt from the care I was able to access there was literally life changing. I can't thank the Tavistock enough for the comprehensive, thorough and sensitive way in which they took care of me. Without the NHS and Tavistock, I wouldn't be the man I am today – in more ways than one, of course. I, and countless other trans people, are eternally grateful for their service, and its closure is a great loss.

Chapter 10

FIRST STEPS – BLOCKERS AND TESTOSTERONE

Gemma

For the next stage of Leo's transition, and where it started to become more physical, we were under the care of Professor Gary Butler, who oversaw all the trans patients as part of the Gender Identity and Development Service (GIDS) clinic run at the Elizabeth Garrett Anderson ward at University College London Hospital. This clinic prescribes and administers puberty-blocking drugs on behalf of the Tavistock's GIDS service. It's a small, friendly clinic that we've now visited many times since Leo's report from Tavistock, and where he was regularly weighed, measured, talked to and with, and had bloods taken. (I'm never any good at that bit and have to leave the room. I am crap at blood tests myself and have fainted in the past, so I can't even think about it. Thank God Leo is a lot braver than me!)

We never actually met with Professor Butler, but the staff on his team were always excellent. Someone from the Tavistock was also always present in the consultations, to ensure a continuity of care between the two arms of the service.

For Leo's first blocker injection, we had to go to UCLH, to the "main" part of the hospital. Leo, Luca and I trooped along and upstairs to a children's ward. We waited outside the main ward area, where there was a mini train and a handful of plastic chairs. Luckily, no one else was waiting, as there wasn't much space! I took a short video of Leo while we waited and asked him, "How do you feel?" in my best journalist voice, thrusting an empty hand toward him as if I was holding a microphone. He replied in his fake deep voice, "Nervous, and excited." He looked a bit sheepish and jittery. We all felt the importance of the moment and what it had taken to get there. Yet, as is often the case, the actual process was so normal and banal. After a while, we were invited back into the ward, and Leo was asked to hop onto a hospital bed. It felt odd being on a main ward just for an injection, and we were feeling a bit on edge and giggly. Someone pulled a curtain around us, and there was also a curtain around the next bed. Luca and I hung around, looking out of the window. Leo was laying on the bed. The day was really warm, and the ward felt hot to me as I stood there holding all our coats. Then, a disembodied voice asked, "Hello, how are you doing today?" Leo answered, "Yes, good thanks," and then we all realized it was a doctor asking the patient in the next bed. We all dissolved into very undignified giggles, made even worse by the fact that we felt like we shouldn't be giggling at all! You know what those situations are like – the very fact that you feel like you can't laugh makes everything instantly funnier. Luca has a very infectious giggle, too, and once I get giggling, I find it hard to stop. It certainly helped dispel the tension we had all been feeling.

A really nice guy soon came along, checked Leo's name and date of birth, and confirmed what he was in for. He gave Leo the jab in his bum – the first of many – and we were done! All that build-up, and then such a momentous occasion was done and dusted in an ordinary five minutes on an anonymous hospital ward. It was all a bit surreal. We wandered back out and went across the road to get some lunch, then went home! Stage one of Leo's "official" and medical transition was ticked off.

Testosterone was the next part of the plan. We knew what was going to happen right from the first meetings at Tavistock –

although blockers were the short-term goal, testosterone was the long-term goal. It was going to be testosterone that started to physically turn Leo into a man. He would get broader, hairier and stronger, and find it easier to build muscle.

So, even though we knew that the goal was to go on testosterone, when the time came and Leo was due to start, it caught me out. We knew that, unlike blockers, where the effect is basically temporary, testosterone was about to start making physical changes to Leo that weren't reversible.

I found that the idea of it was more upsetting the closer we got to that first injection, and I didn't really understand why. I could see how much it meant to Leo – it was basically the most important thing that had ever happened to him. It was nothing but positive for him. He knew there may be some side effects – some sooner (acne, shorter temper) and some later (possible infertility), but his mind was 100 per cent made up, and he was super excited to start.

I wanted to be excited, too, and I had really tried to be a supportive parent. But looking back on this period, I think it's important to realize that you can still be emotionally affected by the things that are happening to your child. It doesn't make you unsupportive – it just means you're a parent dealing with things your child's going through. It was a reminder that it still wasn't going to be that easy.

For Leo's first testosterone injection, we were back again at UCLH, but a couple of years later. As usual, we – Leo, his girlfriend at the time, and I – took the train to the appointment and we were cutting it a bit fine timewise, so we walked at top speed along Euston Road from St Pancras. It was another blustery London day, and we all got a bit sweaty as we raced up Euston Road, shouting to each other and darting in between other pedestrians. We asked at the main reception where to go, and they pointed us to the right ward.

We were shown into a room where Leo was asked to come behind a screen for the injection while I was told to wait outside. His then-girlfriend was allowed behind the screen with Leo, at his request. Now used to yanking his trousers down to hip level for his blocker jabs, Leo had a much better idea of what to expect. Sustanon, the medical version of testosterone, is a bit of a different kettle of fish, though. Dissolved in oil, it is thick and harder to inject. I've seen the needles since that day, and they are bloody massive! I think it's a good job Leo is used to it and that it's going into a fleshy part of his body.

Leo came back from behind the screen with a HUGE smile on his face. Testosterone felt like the culmination of years of planning, talking and thinking about his transition. The blockers were one thing, and had successfully stopped his female puberty and the dreaded periods. But testosterone was the missing link – it was this that was going to start transforming his body into that of a man. The excitement was palpable, and Leo felt on top of the world – so he was easily able to put up with a bit of a tender bum cheek.

He started off with an injection every month. We had been warned about potential side effects, one of which was a quickness to anger, and this is something we definitely noticed with Leo. On a few occasions, we noticed that he seemed to get grumpy quickly, and there were a few sharp retorts in his conversation, which were unlike him. I remember walking into town with him once, and we were chatting about something – or rather, I was chatting and getting monosyllabic replies in return. I asked if I could give him a bit of feedback about something and got a very short reply – "No." Wow. This was not like Leo at all! So, I changed the subject, gave him a bit of space and stopped talking for a bit. It didn't take too long, luckily, before he made some effort to pick up the conversation, and he did later apologize for being moody. All good fun, and a small price to pay in the long run for his transition.

* * *

Leo

Starting hormone-blocker treatments, and then later testosterone, were, prior to top surgery, the two biggest moments for me in my transition. Beginning my process at the Tavistock marked my first steps on the path to the medical intervention and gender-affirming medical care I'd been so desperately needing. After the assessment period at the clinic, my parents and I consented to me beginning hormone blockers. The day itself, much like other things you dream about and build up in your head, was fairly mundane. I was ecstatic, but when a needle was pressed into me, everything was over in a flash. And that was it – I was on hormone blockers.

Unlike testosterone, there are no physical changes that occur when taking puberty blockers. All that happens is that your puberty, and its continuation, is "blocked", or paused, as it makes better sense to say. There was nothing to notice or look out for – it just meant that, from that moment on, my body would stop developing further, and I felt safe from the terrifying and distressing reality of "becoming a woman", as I saw it.

Due to the lack of physical results from taking hormone blockers, they are often described as giving trans or gender-questioning young people a pause, meaning that they allow them the space to think about, and come to terms with or explore, their relationship with their gender and sex assigned at birth. It can allow them to go through this process without having to continue experiencing a puberty that is potentially causing them great distress, or that they may find harmful. If it is the case that a patient taking them comes to the realization that they perhaps aren't trans, or that they don't want to medically transition, then they can come off the treatment, and their puberty will resume. This is something that is largely overlooked when reported on by the media. Instead, it is often noted that there are few long-term studies on the use of puberty blockers, so people are often encouraged to view them as dangerous and with scepticism. But as far as we know, there are no known long-term effects of puberty blockers, and it is widely accepted that the effects are non-permanent. Throughout the two years I spent on them, my bone density was regularly monitored, as this is something that can be negatively affected by the treatment (but not to a worrying degree, and it has never been a cause of concern). Furthermore, because it's a treatment that is only taken for a few years and then stopped, these things return to normal and no longer need to be checked. The controversy around puberty blockers is yet another example of how the media sensationalizes trans issues and attempts to make the realities of trans people's lives so polarizing. They don't talk about the thousands of kids that have been on blockers who are healthy and go on to transition – they talk about the rare case in the US in which a young trans child may be given them. The real, more monotonous nature of medically transitioning doesn't deliver the big story they're after, so they refuse to tell it.

Though I knew I was still too young to start T, being on blockers allowed me to feel more like myself. I could relax and felt at ease that I wasn't going to become more physically feminine, and this allowed me to grow into myself and become a happier teenager. As I grew older, I felt so much more confident. It felt as if every day I settled into myself a little more. (Honestly, this isn't a feeling I've shaken off yet, but I don't really want to.)

I had used men's toilets before, but I started to feel safer and more comfortable in them (though the cleanliness more typical in women's public toilets is something I occasionally miss). That's because I knew no one gave me a second look being in there now. And if there was a urinal free whilst I waited for a cubicle, I knew people just assumed I was a sitter-downer, though this is still an anxiety I experience a bit with toilets today, especially when there's a queue.

Of course, the last milestone was testosterone. That had always been the goal. When I began taking T, it sort of felt like the first day of the rest of my life (not to be dramatic, lol). This feeling came from the painfully long wait I endured before I turned 16 and was therefore allowed to begin treatment. In reality, it was only four years of waiting, but thinking about something every day for four years of your life makes it feel like a bloody long time. Every day I would think about what changes might come first, when my voice would break, and whether I'd be able to grow a decent beard. (Younger Leo would be pleased with my current abilities in this department.) I remember shaving my hairless face every week to try and encourage facial hair to sprout, and I was always on the lookout for new leg hairs. As plenty of trans guys do, I took a short video of me speaking every month to monitor how deep my voice was getting and did this until about a year on T. Sadly, I've since lost these voice-update videos, which Luca is disappointed by because he used to love flitting between them to hear the difference. But when seeing old videos of myself, I do notice how different I sound.

It is the case that you must be on hormone blockers for about a year before you can start hormone replacement therapy (HRT), which for trans guys is testosterone. The purpose is to essentially train your body to stop producing your biological sex hormones. So, for me, the goal was to stop my body from producing oestrogen. After about a year of taking both blockers and testosterone, I was able to stop taking blockers. In that time, I was required to have quite frequent blood tests to see if I was still producing the female hormones (at the amount I would if I was not transitioning). And my understanding is that the body just eventually stops producing them because the female hormones have been suppressed, which is incredible when you think about it.

At age 14 and 15, I was on blockers but still too young to be on hormones, which coincided with all my male friends and peers at school starting to grow up faster. Not in a maturity sense – I think, thankfully, I was ahead of some of them in that regard – but they were growing up in a way I couldn't achieve. Their voices were dropping, they were getting taller than me and some were starting to grow beards. When I'd first joined the school in Year 7, I was one of the tallest in my year, but as the months and years went on, I was being overtaken. I was lucky that I "passed" well and was never misgendered at school – not by accident, anyway, and I suppose to people that didn't know about me, at this point I probably just looked like a late bloomer. But as soon as I noticed this, I couldn't help becoming increasingly acutely aware of it. I couldn't stop myself noticing how tall that boy had got recently, or how much lower his voice was compared to last year. A sense of dysphoria-riddled panic started to set in. I was already practically counting down the days until my 16th birthday, when I could start testosterone. I didn't think it was possible for my desire for testosterone to be any greater, but I seriously couldn't wait.

I was on blockers for two years before I started testosterone. After my 16th birthday in 2019, I was finally able to start this stage of my treatment. I went up to London, as I had to have my first appointment at UCLH with my mum and my girlfriend at the time. I remember that, on the train and tube journeys, I was sweating from nervousness and apprehension, and yet feeling the most excited I ever have in my life. I was ecstatic. The day of my first injection was a massive day. I'd dreamt about it for years, knowing that one day it would happen. To say it was a surreal moment is an understatement. I was so relieved that this was going to be the beginning of my (second) puberty and, in a year or so, I'd start to look so much more like how I had felt for so long. It was an amazing day.

After this first testosterone injection at UCLH, monthly injections happened through my local GP. They start you off with a fairly small dose because they have to mimic what would be happening naturally in an adolescent male. Obviously, when a guy hits puberty, he doesn't experience a full adult dose of testosterone in his system straightaway because that's not how it works. The body starts producing smaller amounts, and in the same way with my injections,

I worked up to a full dose. I think it was probably over six months before I got my first full adult dose. It went up in increments, every jab or every other jab, and my levels were continuously monitored. I started off having them monthly, and that was the same with hormone blockers. To begin with, I was on Sustanon, a brand name for a testosterone injection administered monthly, and then later, when I turned 19, my doctors at UCLH and I decided to transition me onto Nebido, another brand of testosterone injection that you have once every three months. Part of the reason for that was because it's inconvenient going to the GP every fortnight, which is what I was having to do to keep my testosterone at the desired levels. But because my levels were now stable, I could have injections less frequently. It takes a lot of blood tests and appointments. I'm not keen on blood tests, and I can thank my mum for that. But at least I don't faint during them, which she's been known to do.

The first physical differences I noticed on testosterone were that I started getting very light, patchy hairs on my face. Obviously, at the time, I thought they were so much more visible than they were. I see the sorts of pictures I was taking of them, thinking they were bold and clear. I don't even know what I was taking pictures of when I look at those photos now. Around the same time as those were popping up, my legs were getting a bit hairier, especially on my upper legs, where I used to have nothing above my knee, which always looked funny. Also, my voice started to get a bit croakier and it had the occasional break, although the change was not as dramatic right away as I thought it would be. But my voice started to sound a bit different three months into taking T, and it broke properly by the around six- to seven-month mark. It was pretty gradual, and I don't think I realized it would take quite as long as it did. It was mainly just hope, but I thought that in one or two months in I would sound like a man. I learnt that, unfortunately, that's not quite how it goes.

Those were the first few physical things, and then over a longer timescale, there was fat redistribution, a major change that people don't talk about. I would obsessively watch videos about changes from cross-sex hormones and what you could expect to see at one year, and then two years, and then how things progressed over a longer period of time. Fat redistribution just meant that my body fat would migrate from my hips – where it usually sits on women – to make my shape look less feminine and my hips less apparent. This was aided by the fact I was also working out at the time. I think quite a lot of trans guys I used to watch on YouTube did that as well, which obviously really helped with creating the more masculine figure that I wanted. The fat migration alone made my body shape less curvy, which was a pretty big thing for me because I just desperately wanted to have that straighter masculine midsection with wider shoulders. Luckily, aided by working out frequently, this did occur, and it was a huge milestone for me.

Because I was working out quite seriously, about a year into taking testosterone (by then I was about 17), I noticed how much strength I had achieved in a short amount of time. Now I'm working out consistently and have done for years, so the progression doesn't seem very fast anymore, but it was really noticeable in those early months. What wasn't as fast was the facial-hair growth. It wasn't until around the one-year mark that I started to get a fuller beard. I'd started growing sideburns first, but I didn't really get any hair on my chin for quite a long time after that. Even until I was about 20, my beard didn't connect or really look the same as it does now, and I think it will just continue to get stronger with time. But I have noticed, which apparently is common in some cis guys too, that my moustache grows about two times slower than the rest of my facial hair. When I trim my beard, I leave my moustache for another two weeks, just so it looks the same length as everything else because it's so slow. I've got no idea why that is.

Another T-related change that occurred for me, which I had heard people mention before I started but about which I was sceptical, was how difficult it is to cry when you're on testosterone. I've since learnt that this is certainly the case. I experience some sort of restraint, as if my body is physically trying to stop me, when I feel as if I might cry. I noticed the change because whenever something happened that would have made me cry before I was on testosterone, I didn't even tear up anymore. Before T, crying felt easy – when I did it, there wasn't much to do to stop it. If I felt like I going to cry, I always would. But nowadays, it takes a lot more to make tears actually fall and to do more than just well up. It's physically hard to cry, and I do find it odd. I wonder if that's part of the reason men generally tend to cry less, because it's actually harder to do? This could definitely be wrong, but it's something that intrigues me.

Now I've been on T for almost six years. After the two-year mark, nothing else has really changed about me physically (not due to T, anyway), and this fairly typical I think for trans men. My beard has got slightly fuller and is trying its best to grow further up my cheeks, I've got broader and more muscular, but again, that's due to my weightlifting training as well, not solely my continued hormone treatment. Looking in the mirror, I think I sometimes take for granted my appearance now. I forget that every time I see myself, I'm looking at a man that my younger self couldn't wait to see. And when I shave my face or complain about random shoulder hairs I keep finding, I forget how amazing it is that all these things get to even be there.

When I began hormone treatment, I was told that it would be something that, unless I found a reason not to, I'd likely have to keep doing for the rest of my life to maintain the physical changes it created. This is because there is currently no way that we can get our bodies to naturally produce an adequate dose of the cross-sex hormone we are on so that we can stop taking it artificially. Though it sounds like a weird and sort of morbid concept, I've always like the idea of myself as an 80-year-old man, going to the doctor's on a mid-week morning for my T jab. There's something cyclical and comforting about it. I'm sure there are trans people that might feel depressed or conflicted about the notion of being on HRT for the rest of their lives, but for me, this isn't the case.

Chapter 11

CLOTHES

Gemma

Who realized clothes were such an emotive issue? Not me, until suddenly they were with Leo. As a child of the '70s, I grew up wearing what I liked, pretty much. In one of my favourite photos of myself, aged about six or seven, I'm wearing a brown polyester shirt with orange and white spots, which I had paired with a pair of red tartan trousers. Beyond that outfit, I had a green cheesecloth shirt that was a particular favourite. And I wore quite a lot of velour because I liked the feel of it. So, perhaps I was lucky, as I don't remember being made, or even encouraged, to wear anything in particular. And I usually chose my own clothes. Maybe it was just so my parents could tease me in later life about my choices, or maybe they really just weren't worried.

Looking back, clothes were one of the earliest signifiers of how Leo felt about his gender. As I've mentioned, he always dressed as a tomboy, but while he was small, I bought his clothes. I have never liked the excessively "girly" pink, glittery gear, so I was pretty relieved that as Leo got old enough to express a preference, he didn't like them either. Because he got into street dance when he was quite young, he then dressed very much in that style – jeans, trainers, T-shirts, hoodies and a five-panel cap. He wore that for about the next four or five years, in fact.

What I now know was an early indicator of his trans-ness was not just a preference for boy's clothes, which perhaps wasn't unusual given his penchant for dancing, but an absolute aversion to anything that was "girls'" clothing. Even if it was a plain T-shirt, if it was from the girls' section, it was an instant "no". This was a bit frustrating, as I didn't see where the harm was ... it didn't *look* like girls' clothing, so where was the issue? But Leo made his feelings plain through his actions. Anything even slightly girly or bought from the girls' section remained firmly in his drawers. He was desperate to shop at Topman, but I have to say it took long months of awkward, snappy and unhappy conversations about clothes from both of us before I gave in. Even now, I don't really understand why I was so upset about it. I would tell Leo that it didn't matter about him wearing girls' clothes, but I just couldn't get my head around it being okay for him to shop in a boys' shop, for boys' clothes. JD had become just about the only place on the high street where Leo and I could shop together without arguing about something, even though he only looked in the boys' section there, too.

So, our first trip to Topman in Bedford together was a major event. We hadn't planned it, but we were in town together and, as usual, Leo was desperate to go in. So, we did. I felt super awkward, as I was very clearly not the target customer! But the staff were clearly used to young kids going in with their parents, so it wasn't too bad. Of course, as far as Leo was concerned, there wasn't very much that fit him then, as he was really too young for the clothes that were being stocked, even though he was pretty tall for his age. At the time, I just didn't understand that it was enough for him to be in the shop, legitimately looking at boys' clothes. He was being a boy, shopping for clothes – not my daughter shopping for clothes, but my son. I can't remember if we actually bought anything that day. But I do know that pretty much every time we went to town together after that, we went in Topman, to the point where the staff got to know us, and Leo knew the stock pretty much inside out. There were (still are!) very few places to shop for kids' clothes in Bedford, so Topman was an important place for young Leo. It shut down a year or so ago, along with many other shops on the high street in recent years, which is sad. Luckily, Leo discovered Depop in that time, so he started to join the great trend of buying and selling clothes second-hand. Clothes continued to be such an important part of Leo's transition. I guess they have an important role for all of us in projecting the person we want the world to see us as. Perhaps that makes them even more important for trans people than they are for the rest of us.

* * *

Leo

Clothes were something that Mum and I talked – and argued – about a lot in the early period after I came out. For Mum, buying or letting me wear something "too masculine" was hard because it must have felt like telling me that feeling more masculine was okay, which she wasn't yet ready for, even if it was going to make me happier. There were endless arguments and sharp conversations about whether I could go to Topman (why I was so fussed about that bloody shop, I do not know), even if it was by myself or just for a look. Her difficulty in accepting me was preventing her from realizing that, at the end of the day, clothes are just garments and they don't have to relate to gender. Saying this, though, as a young, insecure and pre-transition trans boy, clothes *were* important to me. Wearing men's clothes was affirming – because there was a label stating who they were for, I got to feel and be received by others as male if I was wearing them.

Even as a young child, as parts of Mum's chapters recall, I wanted nothing to do with feminine clothes. The labels, cuts and colours of them would repulse me, and I would be incredibly uncomfortable in them. In a recent conversation I had with my 70-year-old Gramps at a pub, he told me he remembered me wearing a striped blue-and-white dress with sparkly red shoes (what a combo) for my mum's 40th birthday party. I don't remember exactly how we began talking about this memory, but he told me how uncomfortable and frozen he thought I looked as the evening went on, and how he sensed that I just didn't feel right. He told me, "Now, of course, we know why, but at the time I felt sad looking at you and how out of place you seemed." Considering he and I have maybe had a handful of conversations over the years about my transition or childhood in retrospect, I was taken aback and impressed with his thoughtfulness, the empathic deductions he'd made when revisiting that memory, and the fact such a thought crossed his mind at the time. He is clearly more observant and sensitive than I gave him credit for.

As I got older, after socially transitioning and beginning to present in a more masculine way (not that I presented femininely for that long), clothes developed another dimension of importance for me. Due to the fact I was 15 when I went on hormone blockers, I had already experienced a fair amount of female puberty. I did not have a flat chest or an entirely straight figure. I found out about binders through the trans guys I watched on YouTube, and I felt instantly that a binder would be something I would find immensely validating and useful for alleviating my dysphoria. After learning about binders, I remember begging my mum for one and her responding in a way that told me she very much wasn't ready for me to have/do such a thing, because it felt like that was quite a step in the direction of acknowledging my feelings and dysphoria, which she hadn't yet confronted. But seeing trans guys talk about this stuff probably validated how I was feeling. However, this did eventually change, and she allowed me to research them, and I ultimately convinced her to get one for me.

Though for a long time I wore binders, which helped flatten and masculinize the appearance of my chest, clothes also had the purpose of hiding it further. A plain white T-shirt was not something I would've gone out in public wearing in a million years before having top surgery because I would've felt far too exposed. In my mind, it felt that everyone would be able to tell that I didn't have a biologically male chest. For years, it was patterned tops and shirts, multiple layers in winter, often in hotter months too, and baggy hoodies all year round. I wouldn't just feel dysphoric and vulnerable in public, though. Around the house, I rarely wore just a T-shirt – for years I sported a large, black Twenty One Pilots hoodie in order to feel properly covered up. Worry, panic and anxiety over how my chest and figure looked in clothes wouldn't leave me alone when I was public, so I subconsciously developed habits to help combat such feelings. I would often have my hand up my top, pulling it away from my body, and I would continuously reshuffle and pull the top half of my T-shirt away from me, so the fabric was never up against me or closer than I wanted it to be. I would frequently notice my poor posture, but I knew why I was doing it, so I made little attempt to correct it. I only really realized after top surgery just how ingrained and habitual these responses to my chest dysphoria were, as I would still walk around with my hand pulling my T-shirt away from me for a few months post-surgery, and until I trained myself out of it, I would get to experience the bliss and euphoria of getting to say to myself, "Actually, I don't need to do that anymore."

As a trans boy, clothes are one of the ways we make ourselves feel more comfortable, and like fewer people's eyes are on us. They help us feel that we don't look as weird, or things are not as obvious. It has nothing to do with what other people see, which is what outsiders may think is the reason for binding and dressing masculinely – it's not. It's not so you look at me and think I'm a boy – it's so I can look at *myself* and walk around and feel as comfortable as my dysphoria will let me. It's so I can experience a day, evening or hour and not have what my body looks like in this shirt on my mind constantly.

Now, clothes serve almost the opposite function most of the time. I choose the clothes I wear because I like them and because of how I look in them. My clothes make me feel masculine and positive about my body. They are affirming. I get to enjoy feeling the wind blow my top closer to me and notice how it's pressed against my pec, not what was there before. And how the short sleeves of a shirt hug my arms, which no longer makes me feel embarrassed about their "inadequate" shape, "femininity" or size of them, because I've worked hard to build and like them. My relationship with what I wear has changed drastically, along with many other things since transitioning, and it's something I try to never let myself forget or take for granted.

Chapter 12

SURGERY

Gemma

Top surgery – surgery to remove Leo's unwanted breast tissue – was something that I knew Leo had wanted for years. As soon as he went on testosterone, I knew that surgery was the next "big thing" that I'd have to come to terms with. And it took some coming to terms with.

I knew it would make a massive difference to Leo to be able to have surgery because, as I've described, he was always so self-conscious in his clothes and constantly uncomfortable with his body. He'd started wearing a binder pretty early. They are very restrictive, so it felt like I was always nagging Leo to take it off. But it was clear how uncomfortable he was when he did.

So, surgery might be scary, but I could understand why Leo felt it was necessary and I supported him in choosing it, even though I was terrified about it. How could I watch my young, healthy child go into hospital and have an operation? I know that there is a risk with any kind of surgery, and my fear of hospitals didn't help one bit.

Leo had been researching surgeons for a while, though, and followed the results of other trans men online who had been through the same surgery. So, at least he was going into it with his eyes open. And the good thing about the videos he was watching was that they were real and unvarnished, shared by people like Leo who had been through the same procedure he wanted to go through. We knew there were a handful of surgeons who were well known for this type of work, and Leo and I investigated them. Then the other Leo – the son of Richard and Dawn, who we met through Mermaids – went for top surgery with Mr Peter Kneeshaw, a consultant surgeon in Hull. That Leo was really pleased with his results. We decided to make an enquiry. We were in the extremely fortunate position of being able to afford to pay for Leo to have surgery, rather than wait for it through the NHS. This meant he could have surgery earlier, as he couldn't go on the NHS waiting list until he was 18, and even then, it would be some years until he could have surgery. On the other hand, our private healthcare provider, Spire, offered a loan that allowed us to spread the cost over ten months, making it more affordable. It was still just under £8,000 for the procedure though, which was a big commitment for us!

By the time we'd made the enquiry and waited for our first appointment with Mr Kneeshaw, the Covid-19 pandemic had hit, and we had to do an appointment over Zoom. At that time, I had one of those office pods in the garden (I beat the Covid rush for these pods – I was lucky enough to already have bought one), and because I worked from home more often than I worked in the office, we did the call from there. Our appointment was meant to start at 6pm, but Mr Kneeshaw did not log on as promptly as we did. As time went on and he still didn't appear, we started to get a bit worried, and then a bit despondent. We managed to track down an email address for him, but because our appointment was so late in the day, we didn't know if it would be answered. But then, after about 40 minutes of anxious waiting, Mr Kneeshaw joined the call. We were reassured. With his soft northern accent, no-nonsense manner and tired eyes, he apologized and explained simply that he had been held up. He then talked us through the options, asked Leo why he wanted to have the surgery and listened carefully to his answers. He spoke openly about potential risks and also about what sort of results Leo might expect. He made sure I was clear about everything and that I supported Leo, and he gave us confidence that this was the right choice. But to ensure it was, he asked that we also provide him with a psychological report that confirmed Leo was a candidate for the procedure. Mr Kneeshaw said we could choose someone to provide this, or he could put us in touch with someone he had worked with in the past – Dr Amal Beaini, a psychiatrist who used to work at the Leeds Gender Clinic. So, we had another step to take.

The call with Dr Beaini came soon after the initial meeting with Mr Kneeshaw. We were still in the pandemic, so it took place over Zoom again, cramped together in my little office, sharing a screen. Dr Beaini had a gentle humour and old-fashioned glasses that looked like they were straight out of the 1950s, but sharp, penetrating eyes that seemed to be looking deep into you. Maybe I'm just projecting, but I think years of psychiatry probably meant there were very few people who would get anything past him. His questions to Leo were concise and precise, and he listened carefully to Leo's responses – following up quickly with supplementary questions. After about 45 minutes, he seemed to relax a bit. Leo had been his usual honest and eloquent self, and I don't think Dr Beaini had any qualms with recommending him for surgery. We asked a few more questions about the procedure, and he answered clearly. Then, Leo asked him a question about "bottom" surgery. This seems to be the surgery that most people get fixated on because it's the one that changes your genitals, and for a lot of people who don't understand anything about trans people, this is the surgery that "counts" or that means you've "really transitioned". (All bollocks, of course. Some people never have any surgery. It's a very personal choice about a very personal subject.) Anyway, Dr Beaini explained that bottom surgery for a trans man, called phalloplasty, is complicated and can be pretty horrible. There are several different stages and surgeries necessary. Metoidioplasty takes existing genital tissue and makes it longer, turning it into a neophallus. Then a penis has to be created from a roll of tissue harvested from your arm or leg. A whole load of other stuff has to happen depending on what the desired result is, and it is a lengthy and painful process that requires multiple surgeries. He told us an absolute horror story about a trans man who had gone through all these surgeries to have a penis constructed, for one day to find something falling out of the bottom of his jeans while walking along – his penis. It had basically rotted and fallen off. Hideous, and not something that you can erase from your mind easily once you've been told about it! So basically, it's not a case of a simple "sex-change operation", as some people still think. There are also considerations about removing the uterus and /or fallopian tubes for trans men. It's just all a LOT.

The night before Leo's top surgery was just a bit bizarre. It all felt a bit otherworldly and surreal. We drove up to Hull the night before, as Leo had to be at hospital at 7am ready for surgery. It was set to take place the next day, which happened to be two days after his 18th birthday. It must've been one of the most low-key 18th birthday celebrations on record. Covid-19 was still a thing, and Leo had been told to isolate for some days before his surgery. So, when the date for surgery was set, the party we had planned for him was cancelled. He didn't see any of his friends on his birthday, and instead we had a subdued family dinner, just the four of us. It showed me yet again, in case I was ever in doubt, how much this surgery meant to Leo. His view was very much that he could celebrate afterwards, but that he'd been waiting so long for this moment, he didn't want to do anything that would jeopardize it.

The next morning, Bill and Luca left on the school run, and Leo and I took our time having breakfast and coffee before we set off for another trip up north on the A1 motorway. Leo had taken a Covid test at the Spire Cambridge Lea Hospital the week before, which had come back clear. He'd been isolating, and we'd tested again that morning, so we knew we were good to go.

It was a warm and sunny day, and we drove up at a leisurely pace, stopping for a Starbucks on the way (of course!). We were staying at a corporate-type hotel near to the hospital (the hotel turned out to be in the middle of an industrial estate which was a bit weird). There was a pub/bar-type affair downstairs, which was really our only option for dinner. Leo had requested separate rooms so he could try and sleep well the night before, so once we arrived, there wasn't too much to do. We wandered across the road (which was a bit more of a task than it sounded, as we had to navigate quite a busy crossroads on the entrance to the industrial estate, with multiple lanes running in multiple directions and no real paths for pedestrians!) and popped into the Sainsbury's supermarket for some snacks and drinks – fruit, biscuits, water and juice – and some other bits we didn't really need. What is it about travelling that means you're always hungry and always eat about twice as much as you intend?

We went back to my room and ate some snacks, and then decided to go down to the bar and have dinner early while there weren't many people about. I felt a bit weird and disconnected, sitting in a corner under a massive telly that was showing some kind of sport (golf, I think), and trying to keep away from everyone else. The veggie options were not up to much, and I can't remember what we ended up eating, but the whole thing felt disjointed, while we attempted a stilted conversation. I felt like I was overcompensating by trying to be too jolly. We went back to my room and chatted for a bit. I asked Leo how he was feeling, and unsurprisingly he was nervous about what to expect, but also impatient for it to be morning. We ended our evening together by FaceTiming Bill and Luca and showing them round our very basic rooms. Leo then went off to his room to ring his girlfriend, and I tried to read a book. In fact, I ended up re-reading the same few pages over and over and eventually gave up. I texted Leo next door to say goodnight and tell him I loved him, and then I tried to sleep.

In the morning I woke up early, before the alarm, and got ready before I texted Leo to see if he was up. He was. Before surgery, he couldn't eat or drink anything, so he just brought his stuff back to my room, and we got ready to leave. I took a little video of him to ask him how he was feeling. He said he felt like he had a cold and sounded bunged up. But he said he was also excited. Our friend Issy had messaged to check he'd done a poo, which made us chuckle. (Issy's partner Seb had had top surgery with a different surgeon some months before and had given us a pretty good idea of what to expect … which apparently included not being able to have a poo for a few days afterwards. Turned out it was five for Leo.) He promised to do a video update when he came round from anaesthesia and said sarcastically that he "was sure it would make plenty of sense". And then we were off.

It wasn't very far to drive to the hospital, about ten minutes, and we were both pretty quiet. When I pulled into the car park round the back, we were still a few minutes early, so we sat in the car together. Just before 7am, we got out and walked the few steps to the back door where we would be admitted. A lady with a mask on opened the door and checked Leo's name. Then she told me I couldn't come in with him. I was gutted and felt as though I'd had the wind knocked out of me. Leo had only been an adult for two days, and this was a major operation requiring general anaesthetic. But she was firm and wouldn't even let me over the threshold. I know many people put up with much worse during the Covid-19 pandemic, losing loved ones and not being able to be there with them. But I also felt heartbroken. I was handing over my boy and couldn't be with him to reassure him. The tears sprung immediately. Again, it was down to Leo to be the strong one. He gave me a huge hug and said, "It will be all right, Mum. I'll call you as soon as I can." It was as much as I could do to choke out a "love you, speak to you later, good luck". Leo was taken inside, and the door was closed pretty much in my face while I was still standing there. I walked back into the car and just cried and cried. Big, horrible, gulpy, snotty sobs. What was I crying about? Leo really wanted the operation. I wanted him to have it. But being on his own, having never even been to hospital before, felt huge. I felt that yet again I had failed him in some way by not being able to be with him. I felt guilty and scared, and I had probably just let go of the tension that had been building up in the few days up to this point. Once I had calmed down enough, I drove back to the hotel and scurried back to my room to hide my blotchy red face.

I made a cup of herbal tea and tried to read my book for a while. I had brought my laptop with me, thinking I could do a couple of hours work, but I never even opened it. I just watched the clock for a couple of hours. Leo texted me to say he had been checked in, was in a gown and was just waiting, expecting to go in around 10:30am. It made me feel a bit better that he said the nurses were friendly and he seemed to be bearing up better than I was. He texted me one more time to say he was going through in a few minutes. I waited a bit longer and decided to go for a swim in the hotel pool to get rid of some of my restlessness and anxiety. It was quite a nice, big pool and not too busy in the middle of the morning. I swam slow lengths and looked at the clock about every 15 seconds ... or at least that's what it felt like. It was probably the most unrelaxed swim I've ever had. I tried to stay in the pool for about 45 minutes and then went back to my room, showered again and picked up my book again (I couldn't even pretend I was reading it by then). Time ticked by, and I started to go a little bit mad in the hotel room. I called the hospital but couldn't get through to anyone to speak about Leo, although someone did assure me he would call when he came round and was able to. It got to after lunchtime, and I was feeling a bit sick. I decided I would pack up and start on the journey home as I had planned to. Leo was going to be in for a couple of days, so we had decided I would go home and come back to pick him up. The day was dreary and grey. It was drizzling and there was low visibility, so it felt a bit like walking around inside a cloud. I felt wrong to be leaving without hearing from Leo, but

I knew I wouldn't be able to go in and see him, and that I had a three-to-four-hour drive home. I got to the car and started driving away. The Humber Bridge was only about 15 minutes away, and I'd just got onto it when my phone rang through the car ... it was Leo! Thank God. I felt my eyes fill up straight away again. He sounded drunk, but he sounded like himself, and although he didn't make "plenty of sense" as he'd promised, he could at least tell me he was okay, and it had gone well. I was so grateful.

I was driving slowly across the bridge, looking out but not able to see much beyond the huge wires because of the weather and talking to a nonsensical Leo – it really felt like I was in some other weird dimension. But I was so, so happy to hear from him, and it felt like a huge weight had been lifted. He said he was going to rest and we would talk again later. I spent the next few minutes having another sob, then got on with the rest of my homeward journey while dictating texts to everyone via Siri, and having Siri read out all the responses. There were so many people to message and respond to, and the process was so slow – especially because it was done while driving – that it took me over half the journey before I finished. But it was a welcome respite from all the tension I felt prior to and during the surgery, and a chance to be able to share some of the joy and relief that it had gone well.

A few days later I was driving back up the A1 again, this time with Leo's girlfriend, to pick him up from hospital. We had FaceTimed him on the evening of his operation – he seemed okay but sleepy – and we'd been messaging a lot over the couple of days between the procedure and his discharge from hospital. Luca wanted to come with us to pick him up, but it was a school day, and a lot of driving which wasn't always easy for Luca, so just two of us went to get him. I picked up Leo's girlfriend from her house after the Bedford rush hour, and we trundled up the A1. We were both a bit nervous about what to expect when we arrived, but we chatted happily for the long drive, texting Leo to keep him informed of our progress.

When we arrived, Leo was ready and came out of the same door where I had dropped him off a couple of days earlier. It was such a relief to see him and be able to hug him again. He looked a bit of a state and smelled a bit weird too – that post-operative, sweaty and musty smell from not being able to wash for a couple of days. He was in a white robe – the sort you normally see at a spa – but he looked like he'd been to an anti-spa, if such a thing existed! He was heavily bandaged, as you might expect, basically wearing an elastic body brace all around his torso, with a huge wedge of cotton wool down the front of it to soak up any blood and leakage. It was a bit of a reality-check moment. And even worse, in the pockets of his robe were his two drainage bags, full of blood and plasma, complete with tubes that were coming out of holes on each side of his chest. It was a bit grim to say the least. After big hugs and a few tears, Leo got in the car, and we started our homeward journey. We decided to stop early on at a Starbucks and then try and make it home in one go. I have rarely felt so physically protective of Leo – shepherding him carefully out of the car, making sure no one got too close and trying to get him comfortable in seats that weren't made for comfort in the café. Once back in the car, Leo was really tired, so we had a pretty quiet journey back home, during which I drove very carefully but also as fast as I legally could (and sometimes faster) because I just wanted to get him home safely. It was a tiring journey for us all.

Trying to get to sleep after top surgery was pretty impossible. Leo wasn't able to lie flat while he had his bags attached, so even though I'd bought a big V-shaped pillow, we ended up trying to create this mountain of pillows around him to enable him to sleep upright. I think we used every spare pillow in the house, and there were about nine piled all around him: under his arms, behind his back and neck and head. Thank God he was still physically tired, otherwise I think sleep would have been impossible. The pain had started to kick in, too, and he was on super-strong painkillers, but his back just ached. Funnily enough, he didn't experience too much pain from his chest, or even the bags. But the strain of sitting up and being propped up while strapped into a hot, uncomfortable elastic brace was hard for Leo to bear for the first few days, and hard to watch, too. I amazed myself by being able to help him empty his drainage bags – especially as I'm usually useless at stuff like that. But Bill couldn't bear it and again, I guess it's testament to the things you find yourself able to do for your kids when you have to.

After a few days, Leo started to feel a bit better, and one day when it was nice and sunny, we decided to try going for a little walk. We found Bill's "man bag" (an over-the-shoulder leather bag that Bill only ever used on holiday to put all the travelling paperwork in), and Leo put it on along with a button-up shirt and shorts. We then put his drainage bags into Bill's bag, and we were off. We crossed the road and walked maybe 50 yards before Leo said, "No, I can't do this, it's too uncomfortable." So, we turned around and came back home. At least we'd tried.

Three things made a huge difference to Leo being able to feel better. The first was a shower. Not easy to manage with the bags, but being able to wash off the smell, the goo and the experience, and putting on clean clothes, clean cotton wool and a clean brace really helped. The second, against the instructions of his surgeon, but in desperation, was that Leo laid down to sleep. And he actually slept. We had tried to position the bags so they wouldn't pull and were propped up with pillows, but actually I think he was so tired by then that he didn't even move. A decent night's sleep made a world of difference to how he felt. The last thing was that he managed to have a poo five days after his operation – *five days!* I mean, where on earth was he keeping all the food that he'd eaten in that time?! It still remains a mystery. But he literally felt so relieved and so much better afterwards. Am I oversharing? Maybe, but this is pretty much a warts-and-all account, so I'm sure Leo won't mind me talking about that bit.

After a week, Leo and I were back up to Hull again for the big reveal and the drains removal. Honestly, I've never done so many long drives, and they were starting to take their toll on my back, too. We waited outside for Mr Kneeshaw to come in. The appointment started at 4pm, so it meant a late night back for us, but this time felt very different. I came through with Leo, and Mr Kneeshaw's nurse removed the brace, the cotton wool and the bags, and Leo got the first look at his chest. I have the photo of him with the hugest smile on his face ever. His chest looked very red from the stuck-on badges, and the scar line was massive and dark red. But his chest was flat. Really flat. It was the chest of a young man, one he had been waiting literally years for. It was a good moment. Mr Kneeshaw was really chuffed with the result too and said it couldn't have gone any better. We made an appointment for a follow-up in another month and left for home again. This time, the journey was a lot easier.

* * *

Leo

As soon as I knew about top surgery and what it was, I knew that I wanted it, and that I would have it as soon as I could. And that never changed. I had a friend that I mentioned earlier, Leo, who I met through Mermaids and who was a few years older than me. He had top surgery a year or two before I did, so I was lucky to have someone to turn to who could be on the receiving end of all my questions. We went with the same surgeon, Mr Kneeshaw, because I liked Leo's results and had seen other surgeries he had performed, so I knew I would be satisfied with his work. Plus, Mr Kneeshaw had years of experience performing mastectomies on women with breast cancer prior to seeing trans patients. On top of that, Leo had his surgery when he was 17. Kneeshaw was one of the last doctors who would offer gender-affirming treatment to those under 18, and this was another factor that influenced my choice of surgeon. My desperation to have my female chest reconstructed, and to no longer face dysphoria about that part of body, was a burning desire for me and always had been. There was the option of having top surgery on the NHS but, as we all know, the service was and is overwhelmed, and you had to be 18 before you could be put on the years-long waiting list. I'd been waiting so long already, and I felt like I needed to have this done as soon as I could. So, I was very fortunate to be in a position to have the operation privately.

I had my consultation online with Mr Kneeshaw in October 2020. Usually, these appointments are conducted in person, but at that time we were dealing with Covid-19 lockdown restrictions (although it being online wasn't a bad thing, as he is based in Hull, which is an hours-long drive away from us). In that consultation, he asked me about myself and got to know me generally. Unfortunately, I learnt during our call that he had now changed his policy on age, mainly to avoid criticism, so my operation would have to take place after my 18th birthday. I was pleased that we booked it in for the 14th of September – two days after I would turn 18. We also discussed if I had preferences as to the surgical methods he used. I was always grateful that I wasn't well endowed in the chest department – it had always made binding easier and it gave me more options for my top surgery, too. I knew that keyhole surgery was an option for people that were smaller chested, but I was apprehensive about whether I'd be small enough because the guys I'd come across online who'd had keyhole had, in some cases, looked as if they had the chest of a cis male prior to their surgeries. The keyhole surgery is also referred to as "peri areola" because the cuts are made around the nipple to remove the breast tissue. The other type of surgery is double incision, where the cuts are made at the bottom of the chest, similar to a "normal" mastectomy. This means, unlike with keyhole, you are left with visible scars. As I had years prior to my consultation to consider my surgical options, I reached the conclusion that I wouldn't mind having scars and was happy to take Mr Kneeshaw's recommendation on which method he felt would be most appropriate for me and would produce the best results. When discussing this, he politely asked me to show him my chest so he could have a brief look, which I found a bit awkward but also amusing, so I didn't really mind. Plus, it would help him decide which method he thought would be best for me, so you know, it was worth it. We had another consultation in person pre-op to make the final decision. In that meeting, he said to me, "You're pretty small. The only thing is that you have quite low nipple positioning. If we didn't make the incisions, your nipples could end up being very low." I didn't think I'd be happy with that. Also, sometimes when you're just slightly on the bigger side of qualifying for keyhole surgery, you can get excess flaps of skin at the side of your chest, referred to as "dog ears", which didn't sound desirable, so I opted for the double incision.

Before we could go ahead with the surgery, Mr Kneeshaw told me in our Skype consultation that his patients had to be assessed by a private psychiatrist/gender specialist to decide if top surgery would be the "right" step for the individual and whether or not the patient knew the consequences of having the procedure. Without this additional appointment, he would not perform the surgery. To make this step easier, Mr Kneeshaw recommended someone that he had known and worked with for a long time: Dr Amal Beaini from the Leeds Gender Clinic, who had more than 20 years of experience. So, we had a Zoom call with Dr Beaini too. He was a lovely guy, and he asked a multitude of questions about lots of things to do with the surgery and my history. We covered my transition in a lot of detail, from childhood, to when I came out, to what was going on now and my reasons for wanting surgery. I thought he was thorough, and his advice and comments made a lot of sense. He did confirm to Mr Kneeshaw that surgery was the right choice for me.

The last stage was to meet Mr Kneeshaw in Hull to have a pre-op consultation – the one where he decided that double incision was the right procedure for my body – and that was booked in for a couple of months before my 18th birthday. He took some "before" pictures and he explained everything a bit more to me, and made sure I knew about the risks and was still happy to go ahead. My mum came to the consultation with me, so we were able to discuss everything together. My surgery was booked for 14 September 2021, just days after my 18th birthday. So, although I'd originally planned to have a party, in the end we didn't do anything for my birthday because I had to be quarantined to ensure I didn't get Covid-19 or any other illness, which would result in the operation being rescheduled. I just didn't want anything to jeopardize the surgery that I'd waited so long for. So, though it meant my birthday was a tad boring, we made up for it at a later date. And the night before my surgery, Mum and I drove up to Hull, as I had to be at the hospital first thing in the morning.

We stayed in a hotel close to the hospital, and Mum drove us there the next morning, and we said goodbye. The night before was odd and felt so surreal. Though I tried my hardest to get to sleep, it was almost impossible because of how nervous and excited I was. I knew this would be my last night of sleep with the chest I had loathed for many years. The next day, we arrived at the hospital before 7am because my surgery was pencilled in for 8am. I knew that leaving me there was hard for Mum, especially because I'd never ever had gone into surgery before – I'd never really even been in hospital. When I got in, I was handed a gown, which a nurse asked me to put on. When that was done, all that was left to do was wait around in my room. Mr Kneeshaw came in around 8am and said, "Unfortunately we have to push you back." This ended up being only about an hour-long delay, and although I was disappointed, I knew the surgery would still go ahead, so I attempted to keep myself busy. This was difficult, as I couldn't even look at my phone or pay attention to anything else. All I felt was this overwhelming anticipation, so I don't recall these few hours well, but I'm fairly sure they were spent staring out of the hospital room window.

I remember, as it approached 10am, a nurse came in to tell me that Mr Kneeshaw was ready for me. We walked together through the hospital corridor, which was slightly embarrassing in one of those silly hospital gowns, but you know, I had bigger things to worry about. My heart was pounding in my chest, I was so nervous. The nerves didn't come from the notion of finally having top surgery – they were more due to the fact that I knew I was going to go under the knife for the first time in my life. I sort of couldn't believe it was actually going to happen. As we entered the operating room, I felt like I was in a dream. And all of it was so surreal, it's hard to liken to anything. Mr Kneeshaw greeted me and asked me to lay on the table. I shuffled about, to align my head with the cushion, and began to look around the room where I would have my operation. I could see the nurses placing equipment on a table and I tried my hardest not to look at the tools they'd use for the surgery. Mr Kneeshaw was talking to me, telling me, "You'll soon be awake again," and that he was going to put the mask on me if I was ready. I nodded, and I listened to him count down before I was out. The actual surgery doesn't take too long, between one to two hours, but I remember wondering before I went under what sort of time I'd wake up by.

At some point in the late afternoon, I opened my eyes.

Before I even looked around the room or had my eyes open any longer than a few seconds, I picked up my phone and called my mum. I don't really remember much about this because I was still pretty affected by the anaesthetic, and apparently said nothing that remotely made sense. I think, after feeling relief, she found my mumbling rather amusing because I would attempt to talk for a few seconds and then fling my head back and sort of fall asleep again. Mum told me she was going to hang up, and I went straight back to sleep for a few hours. In the evening, I had some scrambled eggs, which I was incredibly happy to receive, as I hadn't eaten since dinner time the day before, so I was starving. And as a man who eats a lot, I was glad to be fed.

I was only in hospital for two nights, but it is very hard to recall much about them. The days were long, even though I'm sure I was asleep for most of the time. I couldn't get up by myself, and for the first night, I had to have my legs strapped into this machine at the end of the bed that periodically squeezed my legs to keep the blood flowing, which made it sort of hard to sleep. I had drains in, which (trigger warning: this bit is so gross) were twisted around in my chest, under the skin. If I pressed down, I could feel them, and they came out of me through two small holes made under my armpits. Their job was to drain the blood and fluids out of my chest, and I had them in for nine days. I was heavily bandaged the first night in hospital. I had to have assistance to go for a wee, and I definitely annoyed the nurses because it felt like I went for a wee every ten minutes – I had to drink so much water to rehydrate myself from the anaesthetic, and I'm weak bladdered anyway.

Doing nothing but recovering was oddly exhausting. I didn't have the energy to watch TV or shows on the laptop that I'd brought with me, so, much like the night and day before I had the operation, I spent my waking hours staring at various things in the room and occasionally calling family and friends. The first day I felt relatively upbeat and as chirpy as I could be, given the fact that I had just been operated on and was coming off the anaesthetic. But the second day was much harder. They gave me painkillers because whatever I was on before felt as if it was wearing off, and everything just really hurt. Everything about my body just felt so weird, like it wasn't mine. I couldn't feel anything and had no sensation of where the incisions had been made, which I expected to be the case. I felt like I'd been hit with a brick when I started moving again.

The day I could go home came, and I was glad to see the back of the hospital. Mr Kneeshaw and a nurse came to do one last check-up and had a peek at my new chest to see how everything was doing – I didn't get to look at this point, though, much to my disappointment. I couldn't walk very well and still had the drains in, which I had to navigate every time I moved.

On the way home from hospital, we stopped at a Starbucks, and that was the first time I went to the toilet by myself. Only then did I realize just how restricted my movement was – even turning my body was so hard. I couldn't lift my arms up as well as before, so even reaching forward to dry my hands was a challenge. I got some odd looks as the people in the café who were obviously wondering, *What the hell happened to this guy?* I remember when we got home after the long drive, I sat straight down on the sofa and cried. It was partly relief that I was home, but it was also exhaustion and pain. I didn't expect to do that. It just sort of came out, which took me and everyone else by surprise. I'm sure there was just a lot of emotion and stuff my body needed to release.

My posture was appalling for the first week after surgery. With the drains in, I had to wear a big bandage/binder around my chest, which had to be tight to keep everything compressed, so it really restricted my back movement. Those first nine days, I had the worst back pain imaginable. It was constant, and no matter how much paracetamol I took, it didn't stop until I began to sleep normally again. It was horrible trying to sleep with the drains in. I wasn't meant to lie down, or sleep on my back or side. The positions I tried to put myself were just ridiculous. But the worst thing was that no matter what I did, my back was constantly curved, so it was just excruciating. I was so glad when that started to go back to normal.

Then, there was the toilet issue. Another thing I didn't particularly realize about anaesthetic was that it gives you constipation. And I'd never had constipation before in my life. I'm someone who gets a bit stressed if I can't go to the toilet, and I never knew that about myself before surgery. And I hadn't even gone the morning of the operation because of how nervous I was. After the surgery, it was so unpleasant because I looked and felt so bloated. In reality, I was starving because I was just trying to recover, but I didn't eat because I was just so constipated – I couldn't go to the loo. I looked so funny with a massive belly. In desperation, we just bought laxatives, and I had never had those before either. Thank God they did the trick, and it was the best I've ever felt. (Apologies for giving too much information, but I would've appreciated knowing this was a side effect beforehand!)

A week or so later, Mum and I drove back to hospital to get my drains taken out. It was again three or so hours in the car to get there, and I was so excited to have them out. They were such a pain and frankly just gross, so I was glad to be saying goodbye to them. And knowing that they were twisted around underneath my skin was horrible. I thought it would be a bit painful having the drains removed, but instead, because everything was so numb – I guess because those areas of my body were in shock or not repaired enough to feel yet – I didn't even know when it was done. Mr Kneeshaw said, "Right, okay, I'm starting." And I couldn't feel a thing, but I was really glad it was over. After Mr Kneeshaw had done that, he began unwrapping my bandage and cutting through the padding, making his way to my chest. It was a bit of a job because of the sheer number of bandages and padding around my body to protect it, so there were a good few minutes of suspense before the big reveal. When he'd removed it all, he looked and told us how happy he was with the results. Then, he told me to stand in front of the mirror to have a look. Seeing myself in the mirror in that moment felt like something out of a film. It was so surreal because it was one of those things I'd imagined and dreamt about for so many years. I don't really know what to liken the feeling to, but it was incredible. I couldn't control the smile pinned on my face – I just stood in the mirror, overwhelmed with euphoria.

I have a video on my phone, which I took not long after I had had my drains taken out, of me putting on a T-shirt by myself for the first time. It was probably nine or ten days post-op. One of the good things about having the operation when you're young is that you can bounce back fairly quickly. Your mobility gets back to normal quicker. So, at day ten, I was still having to wear the big binder, but I could manage to sort of put my arms through a T-shirt and bend my back in the worst way possible to get my head through it, and then shuffle it down my body. It was nice to be able to do that after wearing button-up shirts and dressing gowns all the time.

Before I got the surgery, I had a job in a café, and I was able to go back to work about two or three weeks after the operation. At that point I couldn't reach up to high things and still had limited mobility. No one at work knew what my surgery was for and were polite enough to not ask questions. It was funny – I thought, *You guys have got no idea why I'm so immobile.* But I could only lift my arms straight out in front of me, no higher than that, when I started working again. So, putting plates back on shelves after drying them was a battle, and I had to go on my tiptoes and almost fling the plates using my shoulders to put them back in their place. I'm proud to say there were no plate casualties during these weeks, despite my struggles.

At just over a month post-op, I could put my arms above my head, but it was a real stretch. It took a good seven or eight months before I could put my arms right over my head without it feeling like a pull. It takes a long time for your skin to allow you to stretch fully again, but you have to be careful not to stretch your scars from too much movement too soon. I was advised to use Bio-Oil for about three months to reduce the scarring, and I still use it now sometimes. My scars look so different to how they looked even a year after surgery. I knew they would fade and will continue to do so, but I'm still impressed by the difference between what they looked like a few weeks post-op to now. I saw a picture recently of when they were fresh, and it reminded me how dark and red they were. At around two years post-op, they are purplish and white now, and much less visible. Overall, the healing process has gone really well, which I'm so pleased about. I didn't go back to working out for about five months after surgery, but it was still pretty light stuff initially. I didn't bench press for almost a year after surgery for fear of overdoing it, and I'd been working out regularly for a while by then, so that was hard … but undeniably worth it.

Afterwards, it was so incredible to be able to wear whatever I wanted. I went crazy for white T-shirts because I'd never been able to wear them before. And I told myself, *I'm going to buy them because now I can buy whatever I want*. Before surgery, I'd used physio tape on my chest to keep it flat. It really is pretty bad for you to do, but it just shows what desperate lengths you go to when you're so unhappy with your body. It's fairly well-known that people use tape instead of wearing a binder, but also that it's really not good for your chest because it basically stops the skin from breathing and then scars and pulls the skin when you take it off, leaving bruises and soreness. Mr Kneeshaw told me during my first video consultation with him that if I kept taping like that, it could affect my results, and I could leave permanent marks on my skin. It was a bit of a wakeup call. So, for seven months before surgery, I didn't wear anything on my chest, not even a binder. It was horrible and dysphoric to forgo binding and taping for that long, but that's why I'm so lucky that I was relatively small chested because I could get away with stuff. Still, before my surgery, I constantly wore patterns and baggy shirts because it was just more naturally disguising. So, after surgery, to have absolutely no limit on what I could wear was so weird, but it was so exciting; and to this day, I have a little moment to myself every time I put on a plain white T-shirt.

At a recent exhibition of his, trans artist Chella Man displayed a piece he'd written after having top surgery. It sums up exactly how I reflect on my surgery and what it means to me, so I would like to share an excerpt of it here. It reads:

> I am currently recovering from
> top surgery.
> I feel as if it is not top surgery I am recovering
> from. It is spending years – my entire life –
> in a body I do not connect with.
>
> This is not recovery.
> This is healing.[9]

Chapter 13

BECOMING ADVOCATES

Gemma

As part of our "we made it through" – or at least our "we're *making* it through" – process, both Leo and I were keen to support Mermaids and help with their promotion, as well take part in other projects that promoted trans awareness and advocacy. One of the first things we did was volunteer for a photography project with Charlotte Hadden, an amazing photographer. Charlotte is a fashion and lifestyle photographer who has worked on and with some high-end magazines and press, and she's photographed many famous people, including actors, writers and performers. Her photos are gorgeous and different. As someone who identifies as queer herself, she wanted to do a personal project about transgender youth and was looking for subjects. She came to Bedford to visit us, and we picked her up from the station and took her back to our house. She spent the day with Leo, taking photos in the house and on a walk through the village. The pictures are brilliant. She shared a couple on her main Instagram account, and when she had a few more subjects, she created a new page for the project. We got to know her quite well, and she's been back a couple more times over the years to take more photos of Leo. Today, we're still in touch and feel lucky to know her. She and I were once talking about how she could promote her work on this project and the fact that eventually she'd like to do an exhibition and a book. One thing we did come up with together was the name for the project – *Between*. Sound familiar? I did check with her, and she was okay with us using as the title for this book, too. Have a look at her Instagram at @between_ portraits for incredible photos of Leo and other trans kids.

We also participated in interviews for a number of press stories, some of which came out better than others. I certainly learnt to be more careful about what I said after one piece came out with the massive headline "I thought that I was losing my daughter" – yuck. I did say that, of course, but in the context of dealing with the whole complexity of emotions. In the midst of an interview, you forget that, these days, pretty much everything anyone says can get reduced to a clickbait soundbite.

By far the biggest thing we did, though, was a TV interview with Sky News, which was running a piece about the Tavistock around the time of the Keira Bell case, which unfolded in the autumn of 2019. I don't profess to know all the details of this case, which caused a lot of controversy, but my understanding was that the Tavistock had prescribed puberty blockers to Keira when she was 16, but after some time living as a trans man, Keira decided that this was the wrong decision and wanted to go back, to reverse her decision and de-transition.

It's something that I hear a lot as a reason for not letting kids "decide" to be transgender: they might change their minds later. There are a lot of circumstances in which people change their minds – people who get sterilized, for example, and then want to reverse this to have children. People who get married and say, "'Til death do us part," and then get divorced. People who have plastic surgery and then maybe wish they didn't. I'm not saying it's impossible for people to change their minds – I got divorced after promising to spend my life with someone when I was 21. But to me, how this case was treated in the press seemed very typical of how a lot of transgender issues were – and sadly, still are – treated, in a sensationalist/who's to blame?/kids being "wrong" type way. It feels partly voyeuristic and partly like schadenfreude ... fascinating and horrible for the public at large. And even more horrible to be part of. Leo and I were both pretty unsure about putting ourselves out there because of all the criticism it would no doubt involve. But we both did feel responsible for at least trying to put across a positive story too. Unsurprisingly, most people that Mermaids approached about participating in the interview didn't want to put themselves through that. Andy, who was the press guy at Mermaids, told us that Sky were going to run the story anyway, and if we took part, at least there might be an attempt at balance. So, we said yes.

On the day of the interview, Leo came to meet me at work in Farringdon, and Andy tried to encourage us on Zoom beforehand. He told us what it might be like and what questions to expect, and he tried to help us feel a bit prepared. We were both super nervous. I got a number of texts throughout the day, which confirmed the time and location of the interview, and eventually it was time to get in a cab and go. We wanted to meet somewhere neutral, so we settled on a park nearby. There was just the interviewer from Sky, one production person and a cameraman with a handheld camera. We sat together on a bench and introduced ourselves. Sally from Sky talked through the questions, and we told her what we thought. Then, we did it again with the camera rolling. Leo did bloody brilliantly. He was honest, articulate, heartfelt ... I was so proud of him. I didn't say much and wasn't asked too much, except for one moment when he had explained that if he hadn't transitioned, he didn't think he would be there that day. I was really choked up and had tears in my eyes. Even Sally did at that point too, and she turned to me to say, "You must be very proud." I was so nervous, and it was so tense that a stupid giggle came out as I said, "I am. Very proud." When I eventually watched the interview back – which actually wasn't until 2022 – I was horrified by that bloody giggle. But there you go. Again, the bits that are left in the interview are the ones that make the impact, and my incongruous giggle probably made people think I wasn't taking it seriously.

The interview didn't come out right away, and then, some time in December, we found out that it was going to run the next day. I realized it had aired when I started getting messages from people. (Who knew so many people watched Sky? We didn't have it, so we didn't see the coverage!) Some of the messages were really amazing – it was just lovely to know that some people understood what we had tried to do. But then I started to see the comments coming in. The comments on Twitter were incredible ... I had no idea people could be so vicious. It was truly awful. "Where's the kid's dad? Obviously not on the scene." "She just needs some sense knocking into her." "Poor, confused, exploited child ... not their fault, just been brought up wrong." Someone even accused me of having Munchausen by proxy! It was vitriolic. Hideous. Awful. I wished we'd never done it. We'd been cut against someone who had done the same as Keira Bell – someone who thought they were a trans boy, who went on hormones and then changed their mind. But this person blamed the system and said there weren't enough safeguards in place, said that getting drugs was "too easy". I couldn't believe that either. It was just the opposite of our experience in every way.

Overall, now that I've finally watched the whole thing, I don't think the interview was too bad. They did show a variety of outcomes and seemed to try and present them (I think) without too much judgement. Most of all, though, the interview highlighted the controversy and need for a better outcome for all trans kids – a better, fairer and less contentious system. One where kids could feel protected and supported, whatever their choices. I don't think we're there yet, but even when we are, the world outside that system has a lot of changes to make before trans kids can feel safe in it.

We had a more positive experience when Leo took part in a short video that shared his story, originally produced by a small independent firm and sponsored by a water company. The latter later decided not to release the video, which was a shame, but the documentary makers still released it on YouTube, so it's still online. (If you'd like to look it up, it's titled "Gender Diversity in Schools" by Callum Pearson.) Callum came to our house and filmed Leo during the day at home and at school. I also took part. The school were fantastic in giving their permission for filming, and the headmaster was also interviewed, along with Issy, Leo's English teacher. Issy was absolutely pivotal in Leo's experiences at school – as we've both said already, she was a huge support for him.

The video was a chance for Leo to talk about his own experiences honestly. We weren't cut against anyone else, and there was no underlying motive in producing the film except for sharing our story. If you go and watch the video, you'll also see how incredibly articulate Leo was, even back then. He's 14 in the video and was living as Leo, but he hadn't at that point started any hormone treatment. Because the video was filmed in conjunction with Mermaids, Susie Green, the former CEO, speaks in it, as does another trans activist. Although Leo's story is overwhelmingly positive, and the video (I hope) gives people a sense of hope for the future. The video also includes some stats about trans people, which are part of the reason both Leo and I were okay with taking part. We hoped that by telling our story – one of a normal teenager and parent – that someone watching it might feel encouraged enough to stop hurting themselves or thinking about doing it.

Another public initiative we took part in through Mermaids was a photographic exhibition at the Southbank Centre in London. If at this point you're thinking we were publicity hungry, I can promise you, we really weren't. It was just very hard for the Mermaids team to find trans parents and kids who were willing to participate in this stuff – not because they didn't want to, or believe in it, but because they didn't want to make themselves visible to the inevitable criticism. Leo and I felt that because we had a positive story to tell, and because we felt strong as a family unit and supported by Mermaids, that we could share our stories because it might help others. That meant that when Mermaids put out a call for help with an initiative, we volunteered. The exhibition was called "Transparent Love" (Trans-parent love) and the photographer was Amanda Searle. Amanda did a whole series of portraits of trans kids with their parent(s) for it. The photos are amazing and do a brilliant job of showing the love in the families who took part. Leo and I went to meet Amanda at her house in South London. We walked around the nearby park, took tons of photos inside and outside, and chatted to her over tea. In the end, the photo she chose of us was super simple – standing against a black backdrop with the sun shining through part of her front window. We couldn't attend the opening of the exhibition with the other parents, which was a shame, but we went along with some friends the following day. It was so weird going into such a well-known location and seeing a picture of ourselves on the wall!

A super cool spin-off from the exhibition was when Mermaids managed to get it recreated in miniature in a room at the Houses of Parliament, in Portcullis House, for Members of Parliament to come and see. A private viewing was arranged, and a number of MPs came along to see the photos and meet the kids and parents. One MP, Stephen Doughty, the MP for Cardiff South and Penarth, even gave us a personal, behind-the-scenes tour of the Houses of Parliament as a group, which was really wonderful. We went into the main chamber, which is so much smaller in real life than it looks on TV, and we saw how MPs vote. Stephen was a real history buff and made the tour even more interesting by pointing out Henry VIII's tennis balls in the roof of Westminster Hall. We were allowed to see the Crypt and walk through the underpass from Portcullis House to the House of Commons – it felt exciting and secret, like we were undercover spies. But that was probably my imagination running away with me, driven by my passion for the TV series *Spooks*!

The first time Leo spoke on behalf of Mermaids was at the Lloyds Bank Rainbow Alliance conference on 3 April 2019. On the Mermaids Facebook group, an urgent request went out for a teenage speaker. Their previous speaker had to pull out at short notice, and they were desperate for someone who would be prepared to do it. I spoke to Leo, and he said yes. The theme of the Lloyds conference was "Generations", and it focused on the challenges of being LGBTQ+ through the ages. There were speakers representing older LGBTQ+ people, as well as the editor of the online LGBTQ+ newspaper Pink News, and Mermaids had a speaker representing young people. I think it must have been the Easter holiday because I travelled down to the conference in Brighton with not only Leo, but also Luca too. (We live at the end of the Bedford-Brighton trainline, so all we needed to do was hop on the train at Bedford and hop off at the other end!) We made our way down to the hotel where the conference was held and met the representative from Mermaids, as well as some of the conference organizers, who took Leo off to talk to him about what he would be doing. As we'd arrived not too long before the session in which he was due to speak, we didn't have much hanging around to do. Luca and I sat at a table near the back of the room. We couldn't see Leo all that well, but we felt a bit out of place, so we kept to the side of the room on an empty table.

The main speaker introduced the panel and explained where they had all come from and who they were there representing. Leo was at the end of the line. One by one, the speakers, all adults, talked about who they were, and the organization they spoke on behalf of. Then it was Leo's turn: "Hello everyone. I'm Leo. I'm 15, I'm a female-to-male transgender person. I don't do things like this. I don't belong to any sort of organization. This is the first time I've ever done something like this, so I'm excited about it." Then, he whispered, "That's really all I have to say." There was a huge round of applause, and I was so proud of him. He was sitting on a stage in front of about 300 people and just talking naturally! I'm scared stiff of public speaking, so I thought he did brilliantly well. He participated in the panel, and when it came to audience questions, he had some absolutely amazing comments and feedback, and many of the questions were directed to him. Afterwards, loads of people came to talk to him, and honestly it felt like I was with a celebrity. People were so impressed with him, his maturity and his ability to speak – it was a very special occasion and one I mostly watched through blurry eyes.

Following on from that, Leo and I were invited by Lloyds to participate in the Pride in London Parade that year, where we met some amazing people – Rachel, Om, Anthony and AJ, to name a few. Lloyds really had a brilliant network internally for LGBTQ+ people, and we were really lucky to be able to get a bit more involved with them. Leo spoke at another event at their offices in Barbican, and he was even offered a week's work experience during the summer holidays in their marketing department at the London Wall office, an experience which he really enjoyed. Later on, I also spoke at an event about LGBTQ+ families and took a friend along with me, who was evidently moved by the event and came out as non-binary the next day! That friend is now living as a trans man, post-top surgery and on testosterone, and living very happily with their partner, who supported them throughout their transition.

One other organization that we have to thank for their support – of myself, Leo and Mermaids – is Sage. I used to work at Sage in the global marketing team, working with partners, and again, they had a strong Pride organization that put on events, run by the brilliant ally and advocate Victoria Rowland. I had known Vicky through work, but when she put on an event to celebrate Trans Day of Visibility, she asked me if Leo would participate alongside her close friend and well-known trans activist, Pips Bunce. It was an evening event in our offices at the Shard, and Leo's teacher Issy also came along to support us, too. It was a well-attended event, and Pips spoke powerfully about the prejudice and problems experienced by trans people. Leo spoke about his own experience, and again, I watched him with tears in my eyes through most of it. I know I'm going on about it, but I don't think I was alone in being moved and inspired – lots of people came up to him afterwards to congratulate him and thank him for his honesty. After that, we went for a pizza and crashed out on the train home. Leo was asked back to speak at the same event, this time during the day in 2021. And at his second appearance, it was a very different person that the people from Sage saw – he was no longer a skinny young trans boy, but a confident, broad and bearded young man.

* * *

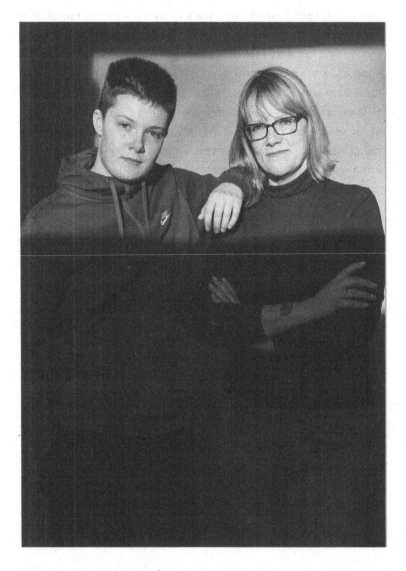

Leo and Gemma, Portrait for *Transparent Love* exhibition, 2019.
Photo: Amanda Searle

Leo

Advocacy is an interesting term when used in this context. The same goes for "activism", because it implies promotion of an issue, which doesn't quite fit the description of what my mum has discussed and recounted in this chapter so far. The word "advocate" could be misinterpreted as us "promoting" some sort of "LGBTQ+ agenda", which ignorant (often right-wing) commentators like to say whenever trans people and allies speak in the media. So, to avoid such criticism, I felt it necessary to discuss in more detail our experience of activism/advocacy for trans rights, and why we participated in such activities.

When approached to do public speaking about my experiences as a trans person, I always feel – and have felt – apprehensive. I am wary of how things can be spun. This was especially an anxiety of mine in the case of the Sky interview that my mum and I did, which, unfortunately, I feel I was right to be worried about. There was a hidden undertone to the video, which I felt was attempting to undermine the decisions of trans children in the UK. As is to be expected, they only included the parts of our interview that were the saddest or most dramatic, and managed to cut the clips together to emphasize that. Meanwhile, they left out the parts in which I discussed how much happier I was after medically transitioning – but I don't know why I was ever surprised by how it turned out. As both of us have briefly and occasionally noted throughout this book, mainstream media today has succeeded in mispresenting, alienating and isolating the trans community in the UK. Though now I realize that I was always going to end up disappointed with the results of that interview with Sky, it's helped me to reinforce why I won't be doing any other such things in a hurry.

In 2019, Mermaids released the findings of exclusive research conducted by Professor Paul Baker of Lancaster University, which looked into news coverage of trans issues. The opening statement of the resulting report reads: "The British press has increased its coverage of stories about trans people over the last six years, writing roughly three-and-a-half times as many articles in 2018–19 compared to 2012." The research found that that not only have trans people been increasingly reported on (over three-and-a-half times more articles in this time frame), but the way in which we are discussed has become increasingly negative. Professor Baker highlighted how trans people are spoken about "in the context of being demanding or aggressive 334 times in 2018–19" (compared to 5 times in 2012).[10] This report captures the tone of the conversation about trans people in the UK today, and shows why, for those who don't know trans people personally or wouldn't consider themselves to be informed and/or an ally, the idea of transgender people can easily be distorted. Is it any wonder that there's pushback from the community, considering the way we are defiled, defamed and undermined so consistently in media and representations? Such evidence alludes to why the public speaking I've done has been in more private, media-free settings, presenting to rooms of people instead of a camera. I feel that what I have to say and share can be best received in this way, instead of putting myself and my parents in a position of potentially being ruthlessly denigrated and criticized in an online comments section beneath an article or video clip. I know of other trans people/figures who feel the same about mainstream media appearances, and I don't think our aversion or apprehension to involvement with it is without justification.

As I hope is clear, my mum's and my involvement in presentations and talks about trans people and my transition has only ever been to inform those who wish to know more and are interested in hearing about a real-life experience. It is for much the same reason that I chose to write this book. In a time in which trans people are being attacked by the media, misunderstood by the public and, in cases around the world, *killed* for who we are, it is crucial to have stories like ours out there. Not because there is anything extraordinary or special about us or my experiences in particular, but because, for people who need it, it's another positive reinforcement of how a life is made better when a trans person has been supported, accepted and allowed to follow the path they chose. Though it's incredibly cliché, if there has been one trans person that has felt hopeful reading this book, or one cis person who feels that they now better understand trans people and what they might go through, then writing it all down has been undeniably worth it.

Chapter 14

WHERE ARE WE NOW?

Gemma

When I first wrote this chapter in September 2022, Leo was a few days away from his 19th birthday and almost a year on from his top surgery. He'd just got his A-level results and did well, although just missed out on the A he was hoping for in sociology (due, we're sure, to the reduction in the number of A grades given out as marks were "normalized" after the Covid-19 pandemic). It was pretty tough for a student who got pretty much straight As in two years of study, and something that definitely took the shine right off results day.

But yet again, Leo's maturity shone through. Although then he was fairly sure that he'd like to go to university, he decided he would wait until he got his grades, then consider where he would like to go and then apply. This meant there wasn't pressure on him to get certain grades in order to make the next step, and that he didn't have to wait to find out if the future he was hoping for could happen. Instead, he took the very pragmatic decision to wait and get a guaranteed place the following year based on his actual results. By then, Leo was working in the café at our local gym. He'd been there just over a year and typically worked around 24–28 hours a week. He was well regarded, liked by his colleagues and customers, and seen as a hard worker.

Earlier that year (2022), he passed his driving test (on the second try, like all the best people, apparently – which I can't quite agree with, having passed the first time myself!). He relished the freedom that having a car brings, and I relished getting my evenings back and not having to pick him up from work at 10 and 11pm! His car – a Corsa, known fondly as "Big Dave", and slightly battered from being reversed into a skip in his first few weeks of driving – lived on the driveway just outside our house. It was great that Leo was able to drive Luca around through the school holidays and that they could go to the gym together too, as Luca was at that point also getting interested in/mildly obsessed with working out. Leo just loves going for a drive … with his mates, with his brother or whoever will go with him. He drives around the villages that I used to drive him around in the evenings, playing his music and chatting. Only the cost of petrol stops him doing it all the time, I think.

During Leo's gap year, the open day university visits came and went, and then in 2023, Leo took up a place to study sociology at the University of East Anglia in Norwich, with a view to teaching it at A level himself. There's no pressure from us to take one path or another – we trust Leo to make the best decision for himself now and in the future. Of course, I was kind of desperate for him not to leave home, as I felt like I'd be losing a part of me and my ally in "doing stuff" (Bill and Luca prefer being at home, whereas Leo's answer on doing something, going somewhere or travelling is always "yes"). But so far, it's been okay. He's come home regularly (and not just with washing!), and we've messaged most days. I do miss him, but I know he's having a great time. The campus feels safe, and Norwich is a lovely city. He's already met some great friends and told some of them about himself – even one or two about this book!

* * *

As I write this section again, now in very early 2024, physically, Leo is quite literally a changed man. He's now over two years on from top surgery. He's been on testosterone for over six years now, and although he's always been interested in working out, the testosterone has definitely helped him. He's much broader in the back and shoulders and is really strong. He could finally do a muscle-up just before his surgery, and although he hasn't tried to do one since, he's hitting new personal bests on the bench and leg press at the gym and feeling better now he's able to get back there regularly. It feels like he's settled into himself.

It really feels like the next stage of his life is getting ready to start. I guess everyone is proud of their kids and feels this mix of emotions as you see them growing up, growing away from you a bit and blossoming into themselves ... becoming adults with their own lives. But with Leo, it feels extra poignant. He really is becoming the adult he's always wanted to be. He looks entirely a man – broad, with a crew cut, but smiley, kind and funny. He's navigated changing his whole life over the last eight years. I am still astonished not only by his bravery, but how he's faced changing himself, his appearance, every aspect of his life, while dealing with the fact that almost everyone he knows (and many people he doesn't) know that he "used to be a girl".

Whatever he chooses to do next, I know he's got the wisdom and the compassion for himself and others to make the right choices. And he's got the strength and courage to face whatever adversity life may bring him, too. He's my son, and I could not love him more or be any prouder of him.

* * *

A NOTE ON BEING STEALTH AND WHAT IT MEANS FOR ME – LEO

For those who aren't aware, which is absolutely to be expected if you don't know much about trans people, "stealth" is a descriptor of those who are living and presenting as cisgender, or cis. In other words, people who are trans but who does not make their transness known to those around them (to varying degrees) are described as being "stealth". The aim for most is to be perceived as cis, usually for the purpose of avoiding the stress, awkward conversations or assumptions being made about you – basically, to escape all the fun things that come with being openly trans! It is more often the case for those who feel they don't "pass" (as cis) well enough, or feel they are at risk of assault and/or hate crimes, that the decision to be stealth and keep their identities private is for safety.

Stonewall's 2018 *LGBT in Britain – Trans Report* found that 41 per cent of trans and non-binary people in Britain had been the victim of a hate crime.[11] Stop Hate UK found that, between 2020–2021, the trans community were the most targeted group within the LGBTQ+ community as a whole, although, sadly, 88 per cent of trans people do not report the hate crimes they experience.[12] In early 2023, 16-year-old trans girl Brianna Ghey was stabbed to death by two of her peers, and it can't be ignored that this was likely a hate crime, or motivated by feelings of animosity about and aversion to the fact she was trans (as evident through the conversations her attackers had about killing her). Even after this horrific attack, the prime minister at the time, Rishi Sunak, felt it acceptable, in the presence of Ghey's mother, to make a transphobic jibe in the House of Commons.[13] These examples alone show that being stealth, for thousands of trans people worldwide, is not a choice, but a survival tactic.

Some trans people, depending on their life circumstances, make the choice to be completely stealth, meaning that, for however long they wish, they keep this very private element of their identity to themselves. This is completely fine, as frankly, someone's transness is very personal. The way transness is openly and overtly discussed in media today seems to make people forget that this is the case. However, it concerns parts of a trans person's life they potentially feel disconnected to/ uncomfortable about, and it may, for the majority, concern their relationships with their bodies and physical transitions. Typically, outside of the context of being trans, it is not common to talk about your body, genitals or sensitive parts of your personal history with those you don't know very well. However, it has become totally normalized *within* the context of being trans, and the usual social rules seem to disappear when meeting or learning about a trans person. People ask what they want and feel they have a right to do so. There have been countless times when the first thing I've been asked after telling someone I'm transgender is if I have a penis or not. In almost no other scenario would someone ask another person about their genitals or what they're planning to do with them.

As I have progressed in my life and transition, the option to be stealth has presented itself increasingly over time. When in school, I had virtually no agency or choice over who I decided to tell or when, because, due to the nature of secondary school, it seemed everyone knew already. Even in Year 11, I would have Year 7s coming up to me asking if it was true that I "used to be a girl". These were kids whose existence I was entirely unaware of, and yet they had come to learn about such a private part of my identity that I felt I was entitled to retain some control over. Clearly, for many years, this wasn't the case, and this was a fact I resented. It was odd being automatically deprived of the privacy I was entitled to.

Though I didn't realize it at the time, I think part of my motivation for leaving my secondary school to join a sixth form elsewhere was so I would have the opportunity to be more stealth than I ever had been. Even though I came to realize in my first year that there were a few students in my sixth form who knew me prior to my social transition and decided this was knowledge to share with their friendship groups, I mainly found that the choice was mine when coming out.

It was a freeing experience. But coming out is always daunting. I tend to only come out to those I feel I have a genuine connection with, or those who I'd like to become closer to/have come good friends with. It's important to highlight that it is never the person that puts pressure on me to come out – it's merely the fact that, if I am fond of someone, I feel they can never get to know me fully if I don't do so. In romantic relationships, I know it is something that will be necessary for them to know eventually, so I just have to pick a time when I'm comfortable enough to share. Still, this doesn't eliminate the fear of a bad reaction. As I've learnt, people can be unpredictable. When meeting people that I become romantically involved with, it can be more anxiety-inducing than usual. I am "lucky" enough that I feel, and am often told (which people think is a compliment), that no one would know about my transness unless they were made aware of the fact. But despite how grateful I am for this, it can make being stealth a lot scarier, as my transness isn't something people expect from me.

Now that I am at university, I have entered another new social space in which I retain privacy over my identity. I have told a few people that I live with and have become good friends with, but I plan to keep it to this minimum, partly because I've never been in an environment where so few people around me know about it and I want to enjoy my adult life without having such things at the forefront of my mind. This isn't to say that if trans issues ever come up in conversation at a pub or in a social situation that I will sit there and pretend I'm clueless – I will defend my community at every opportunity I can. But to know the people around me aren't adjusting their conversations or walking on eggshells around me makes me feel free and gives me the space to feel disconnected from my past, which I think we all desire at times.

Leo

As I write this chapter, I am studying away from home at university. I will be 21 when *Between* is published and in my second year of studying sociology. I am lucky enough to be surrounded by good friends, some of whom have known me prior to, or met me very soon after, my social transition, which makes them a priceless support network.

I certainly feel that I'm at a "transitional" point in my life. Living away from home, learning at a higher level of education and fully entering adulthood are the kind of things children imagine so much that, at times, it all feels quite surreal. In a way, writing this book has helped me feel as if I can close the chapter on my life before now – before I entered adulthood as the man I am today. Not that I will or even want to forget my experiences, but writing about them and looking inwardly has helped me learn that perhaps I still carry some of the hard parts of it with me. Writing has also helped me feel more at peace with what me and my family went through. Looking back on everything through the lens of my current life is something I've found beneficial and valuable.

Transition is a limiting concept. As noted by Mermaids patron Munroe Bergdorf in her book *Transitional*, we all transition in one way or another. Our lives evolve continuously, and for trans people, this occurs in a more unusual way than for others. But it is still something we can all relate to – and something that we all have in common with one another. Beyond that, I feel that I could write this section a hundred times over and keep finding something new to say, or discover a new outlook on something and want to completely alter what I've already written. That is something I am sure of.

I am *not* entirely sure of what I want for myself in the future – which, as I have admitted to myself, is not something I am used to feeling. Especially regarding my transition, I have always known what I've wanted next and how to reach the next step. I knew after hormone blockers that I would pursue HRT and top surgery after that. The same goes for my education. The path for me, in that respect, was slightly less clear, as I didn't decide I wanted to go to university until I started sitting my A-levels, hence the motivation for having a gap year. But as I write this, I am in university and I wonder what's next. It's scary not to have a sense or strong feeling as to where I want my life to go, but the vagueness is something I feel excited about, the more I reflect.

Despite the uncertainty, I'm not afraid of my future because I am entering it as Leo. As I should be.

ACKNOWLEDGEMENTS

Gemma

I read a lot of books. Mostly fiction, but a bunch of other stuff, too. Whenever I finish a book, I always read the acknowledgements. I enjoy seeing the writer "in real life" and hearing about how their book came to life and the people who helped them along the way. With this book, I feel like you've probably got to know Leo and I pretty well. Possibly we've over-shared, but I know when we decided to write this book, we did it from a place of wanting to help other people. We wanted other trans kids and their parents to know that they're not alone. That other people have been through the stuff they're going through – or at least some of it – and that we made it through. That a lot of the hard feelings of guilt, grief, frustration and pain are normal, not shameful (even though they might feel shameful at the time). So, I really hope that for some of those trans people and their families, this book might help them feel seen and understood. I also hope that it's useful for people who just want to know more about what it's really like being trans or having a trans child.

A lot of people I talk to are supportive, but they often preface any question to me with, "I hope it's okay to ask this ..." I always say yes, but also understand that it's common for people to feel so scared of saying the wrong thing that sometimes it's easier not to say anything. So maybe we've been able to answer some questions here for people. If we haven't, I would say this – if you meet trans people, ask them your questions. Most people will be open to talking about things if you ask them if it's okay first and explain that you want to know to be in a better position to support others. For me, being an ally to trans people means taking the time to understand what's going on with them and having empathy with their situation. Trans people seem to be under more pressure and scrutiny than ever these days, and I can only hope that eventually the bigots will get over themselves and crawl back under their nearest rock.

Anyway, there are definitely some people I need to thank who helped, encouraged and inspired me to write this book. My two best friends – Tracey (my Old Same) and Teresa (my bestie) – have both spent years encouraging me to write. They've bought me books to write in and always believed in me. Clare, my MA course lead, was always super encouraging and positive about my capabilities. My parents, especially my mum, always encouraged me, and my mum was also an early role model of a successful woman working largely in a man's world.

I had been writing some of this book for the last few years, and then it was at a lunch with my Monday Night Art Club gang that Pat, one of the people I'd been sitting beside in classes, talked to me about Leo. I knew Pat had published her own books and I'd read and loved them. When I told her, sheepishly, that I was trying to write a book with Leo, she was not just encouraging in the normal sense – she really gave a me a feeling that our book needed to be written and would be important and valuable. More than that, she then spent time with me talking about how to write a book proposal for a non-fiction book and bought me a copy of the *Writers' & Artists' Yearbook*, which was an invaluable resource. Then, when I sent her the book proposal, she was so positive and she also shared it with her daughter, Kate, a literary agent. So, it's largely thanks to Pat that I actually got off my backside and made a positive move to get this book written! I also shared the proposal with Clare (again!), Teresa, and my coach and mentor Roger, as well with Issy, a friend and English teacher you might remember – they all made tons of positive and helpful comments. So, thank you to all of you!

Thank you to Andrew James from Frog Literary Agency for introducing us to Soraya from Trigger Publishing, who Leo and I just clicked with right from the start. And Soraya, thank you for believing in us and our story and helping us to get it out there! Alex – thank you so much for our brilliant author photos and for being so patient with us while we just fidgeted and chatted! To Amanda, whose photo from the Transparent Love exhibition we have shared here with her permission, thank you. And to Charlotte, who has taken many photos of Leo that, in the end, we didn't include here – not because they aren't brilliant, but because we weren't sure how helpful amazing photos of Leo would be to others who might be struggling – thank you, too, for being an advocate and a friend. Thanks to both of you, not just for the brilliant photos of us, but of your work in raising awareness around transgender issues through your photography. xx

But of course, it's my family who really allowed this book to happen. Without Bill by my side these 20-odd years, and through the difficult times described in this book, and otherwise through rough and smooth, I don't think I would have even considered writing it. Luca, despite being a bit concerned about what the ramifications of writing this book would be, has done nothing but support Leo his whole life, and has graciously agreed to let us talk about him a bit. I don't just have one amazing son – I have two. And my love for Leo never means there is less for you, Lulu. To the rest of my family – my little bruv, Piersy, Niki, my stepsons, Mikey and Aaron, and Daisy the Queen (the world's best English Bull Terrier), you all matter so much to me.

And, of course, to the one I really couldn't have written this without: Leo. Bro, I think we both know what writing this book has meant, but to be your mum makes me so unbelievably proud. Your strength in these times that we've gone back and written about – the hardest times I've think we've ever been through – amazes me.

I know you were often there for me in a way that I wasn't for you, and I am so bloody grateful for that, and for your forgiveness. You are an extraordinary person, and anyone who gets to have you in their life, has a better life because you are in it. I still think you should be prime minister. Love you. xxx

* * *

Leo

Between has long been an idea of ours. It was something my mum and I spoke about often, but as if it was something we'd forever dream of that didn't, for me at least, feel likely to really happen. Not because I didn't want it to, but because I thought it would remain one of those things you never get round to. We would discuss it on walks together – our ideas for different chapters, the impact it could have on people – but it wasn't until years later that we sat down and started writing. I am so happy we did get round to it. Writing this book and having the opportunity to share our story has been a pleasure, a privilege and an important journey for me personally. It has allowed me to recount and look back on such a tumultuous but crucial part of my life through a different lens, which I've found hugely valuable.

I would like to thank our agent, Andrew, and our commissioning editor, Soraya from Trigger Publishing, for making this possible, and for making our long-standing idea become a reality. Their support and belief in the book have been integral.

As readers will have picked up on, there were teachers in my secondary school who stuck up for me and provided sanctuary for me when I felt I could not escape from what I was enduring. If there's a chance they are reading this, then they will know who they are. Please know I am so grateful for your support. Thank you to Issy, who kindly looked over our early book proposal and offered her valuable and greatly appreciated insight (and thank you for letting me cry in your classroom endless times xxx).

I could not have got through many of the hard times I've described in this book without my best friends, and I would like to acknowledge their importance in my life. Sam and Harry, I have already told you how much I love and appreciate you. Maddy, your presence in my life is something I am continuously grateful for. You have always been an amazing friend and someone whose opinion I value greatly. To all my friends, thank you for always being there, I love you so much. I will never be able to tell you how much I appreciate your love, company and support.

My brothers have been by my side throughout my life and transition, and I couldn't do without them. Thank you to Luca especially for being my first support and experience of acceptance – you know how much you mean to me, Lulu.

Daniel, you have been so important to me in ways I don't think you understand. Thank you for being so amazing and supportive, and the most gorgeous man I've ever set eyes on. I love you, Mr.

To my amazing father – though we went through much of what this book has discussed separately, it hasn't changed the fact I always have looked up to you. Your ability to adapt and support me to the extent you do is something I am in awe of you for. I love you. And never forget that I can beat you in an arm wrestle these days.

Bro (Mum), I am so proud to have written this with you. You are my inspiration and greatest supporter. I am so lucky to have the relationship I do with you, though I don't think it would be what it is without all we've gone through together. Thank you for all you do and have done for me. I wouldn't be the person I am today without you. Love you too. xxx

I feel it's important to highlight that, though my transition in all aspects hasn't been easy, my background and family's position has made it a hell of a lot easier. Trans people generally are more likely to live in poverty at elevated rates (this is higher amongst trans people of colour), and suffer homelessness and rejection from their families. Without the privilege and resources my family and I have, my transition would not have happened the way it has, and I would've been unable to access surgical intervention when I did. These are reasons that access to trans healthcare and legislation surrounding trans people must improve. It is paramount that governments globally work to ensure our lives and identities are protected properly.

Therefore, lastly, I would like to acknowledge trans people everywhere. Though I don't know many personally, which has always bothered me, it is a part of myself I am so proud to share with so many others around the world. In the face of adversity, discrimination and hostility, we can take solace in the fact that, regardless of geographical boundaries, we are not alone. We must continue to campaign and fight for the improvements and recognition that we deserve to achieve. I hope this book has been valuable to its readers, and that we've been able to provide an insight into what it can be like to come out, parent a trans person, and live as a trans person in the world today.

Thank you for reading.

REFERENCES

1. Faye, S. (30 March 2018). Trans visibility is greater than ever – but that's a double-edged sword. *The Guardian*. Available at: https://www.theguardian.com/commentisfree/2018/mar/30/transgender-acceptance-media-international-day-visibility

2. Barton, C. (16 January 2023). 2021 census: What do we know about the LGBT+ population? House of Commons Library. Available at: https://commonslibrary.parliament.uk/2021-census-what-do-we-know-about-the-lgbt-population/

3. Department for Education. (2023). Gender Questioning Children: Non-statutory guidance for schools and colleges in England. Available at: https://consult.education.gov.uk/equalities-political-impartiality-anti-bullying-team/gender-questioning-children-proposed-guidance/supporting_documents/Gender%20Questioning%20Children%20%20nonstatutory%20guidance.pdf

4. Saunders, C. L., Berner, A., Lund, J., Mason, A. M., Oakes-Monger, T., Roberts, M., Smith, J., & Duschinsky, R. (2023). Demographic characteristics, long-term health conditions and healthcare experiences of 6333 trans and non-binary adults in England: nationally representative evidence from the 2021 GP Patient Survey. *BMJ Open*, *13*, Article 2. Available at: https://doi.org/10.1136/bmjopen-2022-068099

5. Bell, K. (7 April 2021). Keira Bell: My Story. Available at: https://www.persuasion.community/p/keira-bell-my-story

6. GenderGP. (13 January 2023). New Survey Confirms Bell v Tavistock Case Negatively Impacted Trans Children's Mental Health. Available at: https://www.gendergp.com/bell-v-tavistock-case-negatively-impacted-trans-kids-study-shows/

7. GenderGP. (5 July 2024). Detransition Facts and Statistics: Challenging the Myths Around Detransitioners. Available at: https://www.gendergp.com/detransition-facts/

8. Brooks, L. (19 January 2023). 'A contentious place': the inside story of Tavistock's NHS gender identity clinic. *The Guardian*. Available at: https://www.theguardian.com/society/2023/jan/19/a-contentious-place-the-inside-story-of-tavistocks-nhs-gender-identity-clinic

9. Man, C. (17 January 2018). MAN-MADE: I Just Had Top Surgery, and My Scars Are Beautiful. Available at: https://www.them.us/story/i-just-had-top-surgery-and-my-scars-are-beautiful

10. Mermaids UK. (18 November 2019). EXCLUSIVE: Mermaids' research into newspaper coverage on trans issues. Available at: https://mermaidsuk.org.uk/news/exclusive-mermaids-research-into-newspaper-coverage-on-trans-issues/

11. Bachmann, C.L., & Gooch, B. (2018). LGBT in Britain: Trans Report. Stonewall. Available at: https://www.stonewall.org.uk/resources/lgbt-britain-trans-report-2018

12. Stop Hate UK. (n.d.). About Hate Crime: Transgender Hate. Available at: https://www.stophateuk.org/about-hate-crime/transgender-hate/

13. Grunewald, Z., & Devlin, K. (8 February 2024) Uproar over Rishi Sunak's crass trans jibe as Brianna Ghey's mother visits Commons. *The Independent*. Available at: https://www.the-independent.com/news/uk/politics/rishi-sunak-trans-joke-brianna-ghey-mother-b2492095.html

TRIGGERHUB IS ONE OF THE MOST ELITE AND SCIENTIFICALLY PROVEN FORMS OF MENTAL HEALTH INTERVENTION

Trigger Publishing is the leading independent mental health and wellbeing publisher in the UK and US. Our collection of bibliotherapeutic books and the power of lived experience change lives forever. Our courageous authors' lived experiences and the power of their stories are scientifically endorsed by independent federal, state and privately funded research in the US. These stories are intrinsic elements in reducing stigma, making those with poor mental health feel less alone, giving them the privacy they need to heal, ensuring they are guided by the essential steps to kick-start their own journeys to recovery, and providing hope and inspiration when they need it most.

Clinical and scientific research conducted by assistant professor Dr Kristin Kosyluk and her highly acclaimed team in the Department of Mental Health Law & Policy at the University of South Florida (USF), as well as complementary research by her peers across the US, has independently verified the power of lived experience as a core component in achieving mental health prosperity. Their findings categorically confirm lived experience as a leading method in treating those struggling with poor mental health by significantly reducing stigma and the time it takes for them to seek help, self-help or signposting if they are struggling.

Delivered through TriggerHub, our unique online portal and smartphone app, we make our library of bibliotherapeutic titles and other vital resources accessible to individuals and organizations anywhere, at any time and with complete privacy, a crucial element of recovery. As such, TriggerHub is the primary recommendation across the UK and US for the delivery of lived experiences.

At Trigger Publishing and TriggerHub, we proudly lead the way in making the unseen become seen. We are dedicated to humanizing mental health, breaking stigma and challenging outdated societal values to create real action and impact. Find out more about our world-leading work with lived experience and bibliotherapy via triggerhub.com, or by joining us on:

🐦 @triggerhub_
👍 @triggerhub.org
📷 @triggerhub_

Dr Kristin Kosyluk, PhD, is an assistant professor in the Department of Mental Health Law & Policy at USF, a faculty affiliate of the Louis de la Parte Florida Mental Health Institute, and director of the STigma Action Research (STAR) Lab. Find out more about Dr Kristin Kosyluk, her team and their work by visiting:

USF Department of Mental Health Law & Policy:
www.usf.edu/cbcs/mhlp/index.aspx

USF College of Behavioral and Community Sciences:
www.usf.edu/cbcs/index.aspx

STAR Lab: www.usf.edu/cbcs/mhlp/centers/star-lab/

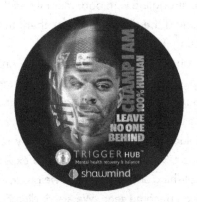

For more information, visit BJ-Super7.com